2019

For bea~ 2

With love

my kitchen to yours.

Brightest

blessings,

Veronika

xx

Love From My
KITCHEN

Gluten-free vegan recipes from the heart

By Veronika Sophia Robinson

Starflower Press

© Written by Veronika Sophia Robinson
© Cover illustration by Tracy Jane Roper
ISBN 978-0-9931586-5-0

Published by Starflower Press - Summer 2017
www.starflowerpress.com

British Library Cataloguing in Publication Data.
A catalogue record for this book is available from the
British Library.

Dedicated to

Pamela Ann Mahoney
25th July 1966 – 25th December 2016

In memory of the long walks, and endless conversations, and the many meals we shared during our eighteen years of friendship, including the Christmases where you dined around our table with us.

The last meal we shared together was on December 16th, 2016. I'd made you red lentil soup in the hope of nourishing you both physically and emotionally. As we sat together in your conservatory, on that bitterly cold Winter's day, I held both your hands and then said a short prayer:

> *Thank you for the food before us*
> *Thank you for the friend beside us*
> *Thank you for the love within us*
> *Amen*

I know my words reached you, my friend, for I saw the tears in your eyes. You will live forever in my heart.

I'm so deeply sorry that I couldn't do more to make you feel this world was a beautiful, loving, nurturing and abundant place.

I will always love you, Pam, across time, space and lifetimes.

Contents

From My Kitchen To Yours

*"When you want to eat,
just spread this magic cloth and you will eat forever."*
Old Folk Tale

Welcome! Please, come on into my kitchen. Will you join me for a mug of vanilla chai tea?

Take a look around (I love looking in other people's homes!), and you'll see glass bowls with beans and legumes soaking in water. Woven baskets laden with earthy nourishing root vegetables, and glass bowls piled high with colourful ripe fruits, will catch your eye. Kilner jars are brimming with life-giving seeds, grains and nuts: snow-white desiccated coconut, sunshine-yellow polenta, calico quinoa, midnight-black beans, red lentils, forest-green pumpkin seeds, and so on.

Old glass jars with wildflowers, and blossoms from the garden, reside on shelves and benches. The radio is set to classical music. Sunshine streams in through the back door, as do birdsong and the joyous sound of children's laughter from the village playground next door.

If there's anything I've learned about cooking, it is this: it's important, if food is to taste great and nourish the eater, that you clear the energetic field around you before you begin food preparation. This means you'll need to breathe deeply, and let go of any tensions within you. When we cook with love, we infuse our food with Divine or Cosmic energy. Eating is an important ritual in the art of living. Do we come to the table with reverence and mindfulness? Is our heart brimming with gratitude for the abundance before us? Or, are we more likely to become unconscious as we shovel food into our mouth? Are we numbing some emotional discomfort?

When I serve food from my kitchen, I'm not just handing you a collection of ingredients that have been combined in a certain way. I'm giving you love. Perhaps you could say I'm recycling the love given to me by The Breathmaker. My desire is not just to fill your hungry tummy, but to nourish your senses and to share pleasure.

"Love" is what I'm sharing with you from my kitchen, and food is Universal Love distilled into an edible form: the foundation for survival on this Earth.

Amongst my greatest joys are walking barefoot in my garden, sunshine on my skin, birdsong in my ear, plucking berries or gathering scented herbs. My reverence for Nature is infused in my love of sharing good food. I was blessed with an earth mother who fed us wholefoods, and filled our plates with fresh, vibrant produce. This template for optimal nutrition is the foundation of my cooking life.

I hope my words provide you with images, and that these prompt your desire to try a recipe and make it your own. You can find photos of many of the recipes in this book on my social media: Pinterest, Twitter, Instagram and Facebook's Love From My Kitchen. Please share photos of meals you've made from this book with me on these accounts. I'd love to see them!

My hesitation when writing Love From My Kitchen was that it would be, like my first recipe book, The Mystic Cookfire, more than just recipes. That it would grow into something much bigger. Perhaps that's why I put it off for so long despite constant requests for recipe book number two. But the simple truth is that food is more than fuel. We truly are what we eat, and the more we can embrace the distilled elements of fire, earth, air and water, then the greater our ability to absorb the nutrients we imbibe, and be truly nourished. We become conscious eaters.

I offer you Love From My Kitchen as a gift from my heart. May the esoteric wisdom my mother instilled into my barefoot childhood come alive in your kitchen with meals which nourish you and your loved ones. I hope that before you skip to the recipes you'll take a few moments to understand why I believe bringing consciousness of the four elements can transform your cooking and eating.

When I wrote The Mystic Cookfire, it was based on my way of eating: a wholefood, plant-based lifestyle. The significant change in my life since then is that I no longer eat gluten, and I rarely use refined sugar as a sweetener in my baking. I do use coconut sugar from time to time, and maple or date syrup.

This book is a distillation of food as a nurturing and sacred art: a story that has been told since humans first walked the Earth.

Life is meant to be enjoyed. Pleasure is our birthright. May you find pleasure in these pages, and make the recipes your own.

If you've read a copy of The Mystic Cookfire, then you'll know you have my full blessing to write notes and leaving cooking stains on every page!

Veronika Sophia Robinson

Eden Valley, Cumbria, England
June 21st, 2017 - Summer Solstice
Moon in Taurus, Venus in Taurus

Why Are We So Hungry?

For many years, I was an active voice in the holistic and conscious-parenting movement, educating families about the importance of our biological needs. At the core of my work, was one word: nurturing.

At birth, when a baby comes to his mother's arms it has five distinct needs. These are all met through the biologically optimal way of feeding a human infant: mother's breast milk (directly from her breast). What happens when these needs aren't met, generally because of routine hospital-birth practices, is that the infant becomes the child who becomes the adult who is always looking for something more. We're searching for the nurturing that comes from breastfeeding in our mother's arms, on cue. One of the harshest parenting practices is that of on-demand or timed feeding. An infant's stomach is tiny. It fills quickly, and it empties quickly. Hunger is excruciatingly painful.

At this preverbal time in our lives, we're always forming beliefs about the world around us. Food, in mother's loving arms, is such a fundamental need for a human, that not receiving it as and when our body requires it in infancy means that we'll never be truly satisfied by any food, drink or oral habit (such as smoking) later on in life. If the synapses in our brain weren't lit up by having our needs met, they die away and the neural pathway ceases to exist. This is a biological fact and isn't said to induce guilt in those who've not breastfed.

Breast milk is liquid love, and is the highest vibration

food we can hope to receive. Once weaned (assuming we had the benefit of any breast milk at all), we can find other high-vibration foods in the plant kingdom.

Consuming these foods will raise your energetic resonance to a higher and healthier emotional and mental frequency; however, your whole life must be lived in accord with this type of energy to match, or you will always feel hungry for something more. The thoughts we think on a daily basis are as much a food and tonic (or toxic poison) as any of the foods we eat or beverages we drink.

Wildcrafted and home-grown food always carry the highest energy, as opposed to foods that are mass produced. The biochemical and spiritual quality of a food feeds your body in a way that's completely different to that which we understand by vitamins and minerals. Each mouthful of food is 'vibrational'. So, while it is good to be mindful of nutrients, being conscious of choosing high-vibrational foods will lead you to optimal nutrition.

After our mother's milk, algae and sprouts have the highest vibration, followed closely by fruit, then leaves and root vegetables. The highest vibrational 'foods' for the human body, however, are pure water and sunlight.

"Preach not to others what they should eat,
but eat as becomes you, and be silent."
Epictetus

Ancient Wisdom

The ancients discovered that the Earth is made of four elements, and that these vital forces make up our natural world: fire, earth, air, and water. By consciously embracing them, and ensuring we have a balance of each in our lives, it means that we not only enrich our body, but enliven our mind and emotions.

Fire *warms*
Earth *stabilises*
Air *rises*
Water *merges*

We see this in Nature, and we see it in how a person who is natally strong in these elements in their astrological birth chart relates to others and the world. On an energetic level, we need:

Fire: *to move*
Earth: *to be*
Air: *to think*
Water: *to feel*

Children of the Moon
The Moon moves through a different zodiac sign every couple of days. Each sign represents a different element: fire, earth, air or water; and each element supports a different aspect of plant life. By consciously working with these energies, our gardens become more prolific.

I'm both a second-generation Moon gardener and astrologer, and am thankful for having learnt this way of being attuned to the heavens and Earth at an early age. For me, the way we move through our garden is a good indication of how we prepare and serve food from our kitchen.

What can the garden teach us? When we eat food, we are, ideally, nourishing ourselves at the deepest level. We are going beyond vitamins and minerals, and seeking sustenance from the elements so we can nurture mind, body and soul.

I am a firm believer that the body *always* wants to heal itself, and that diseases and ailments can be treated by Mother Earth's bounty and beauty. The closer the food we eat is to its natural state, and the happier our thoughts, the healthier we will be.

Gardening by the Moon makes sense. We know the power of the Moon to pull tides, and govern a woman's menstrual cycle. The Moon affects plants, too, because it draws water up from the soil right into the roots, leaves, fruits (including seeds) and flowers. When considering my goal for this book, I realised that these four parts of a plant, and indeed the four elements, would outline my vision.

Planting & Eating
by the Four Elements

Fire *glows*
Earth *grows*
Air *blows*
Water *flows*
Spirit *knows*

When I plant seeds or seedlings, weed or hoe the garden, I do so according to the zodiac sign that the Moon is currently transiting, and the type of plants it impacts most strongly.

Fire signs (Aries, Leo and Sagittarius) rule 'fruit'. Fruit, in gardening terms, covers anything that can be plucked, such as an apple, grain, seed, or pumpkin, for example.

Earth signs (Taurus, Virgo and Capricorn) rule root vegetables; anything that grows underground, such as carrot, onion, leek, parsnip, beetroot, fennel bulb.

Air signs (Gemini, Libra and Aquarius) rule flowers, whether that's a flower for eating or for display.

Water signs (Cancer, Scorpio and Pisces) rule leaves: anything you grow that you want for harvesting leaves.

One way of enhancing your consciousness about the four elements is to choose a recipe that is high in the element that the Moon is transiting that day. So, for example, a water-element day would feature a large quantity of leaves, whereas a fire-element day might feature beans or berries.

Fire *transforms us*
Earth *heals us*
Air *moves us*
Water *shapes us*

Fire and Fruit

"Set your life on fire,
seek those who fan your flames."
Rumi

One of my earliest childhood memories happened when I was about five. My father worked in Papua and New Guinea leading 2,000 men in mining explorations. He was an extraordinary man: pioneering, brave and adventurous. High up in the moist tropical jungles, he led an interesting life. One day, however, a hut caught on fire, and my father ran in to save the family, putting his life at risk. When he returned to Australia with third-degree burns, his injuries were so horrific that I wasn't allowed to see him for weeks.

I was maybe about nine years old when the mountains all around my childhood home in rural Australia burnt... razing everything to the ground. Walking amongst the devastating loss of plant and animal life, I was left with an overwhelming urge to put my feelings into words. It was at this point, I knew I wanted to be a writer. That I needed to be a writer. To, essentially, 'experience life twice', as Anaïs Nin once wrote.

However, fire wasn't just a devastating influence in my childhood, but a fun one, too. Growing up on 700 acres, we would periodically make huge bonfires by gathering up old branches that had come down in storms. Eucalyptus-scented woodsmoke will be forever etched into my heart.

As a young woman, I embraced firewalking on two different occasions. I was living at the Peace Research Institute in the Adelaide Hills, and was fortunate enough to be there when firewalking workshops were held in the elm forest just outside my mezzanine flat. It's quite something to overcome one's belief that you'll be burnt, and just walk across the coals anyway. It was, indeed, one of the most empowering events of my life. To know my mind was so strong truly transformed me, for I knew that if I could walk on hot coals, then I could do virtually anything!

These days, I'm quite content with having my fire contained: the gentle flame of a candle or the way I tend to both of my woodstoves in Winter. Fire warms me, but does not traumatise me. And then, there's the greatest fire of all: The Sun. Oh how I love a hot, sunny day! It nourishes me right to the bones.

Throughout human history, we've been aware that although fire can warm us, and keep us safe, it is also unpredictable and combustible. A small candle flame can become an inferno causing immense devastation. At the time of writing, my eldest brother, Wolfgang, has been actively involved as a Senior Field Operator for the State Emergency Service helping in the aftermath of ferocious and devastating bushfires in Australia.

In some cultures, fire is also used at the end of life for cremation. As a celebrant who officiates funerals, my closing words at a cremation ceremony generally mention that we now lovingly commit the deceased's body to the purifying fire.

Fire is regularly used in ritual and ceremony, such as candles, fire pits, lanterns, firewalking and, of course, cooking. When I lived in New Zealand, I had the pleasure of enjoying root vegetables and leaves cooked in a Māori hāngī. It's a traditional method of cooking food in a pit oven, and uses buried heated rocks.

In psychological astrology, fire signs express the life principles of warmth, radiance, and energy. We see this expressed primarily as faith, passion, drive, enthusiasm, and ability to encourage others.

People with planets in fire signs can 'ignite' easily, too. They're known for their dramatic flair and temperamental nature. Is this bad? When such people express their 'fire' consciously, their passion has the ability to truly light up the world.

Both volatile and passionate, such people can learn not to exterminate everyone they see but instead use their burning energy to make the world a brighter place.

I know from my experience of bushfires, that fire is designed, by its nature, to spread. It's an impulsive energy that defies any boundaries. Those with this strong in their natal chart may be inclined to act before thinking. The key words of the fire energy in the astrology chart are light, anger, passion, Yang, radiate, morality. It's also about learning to love, and vibrancy.

In my native Australia, there is a remarkable plant called the Sturt Desert Pea. It produces incredible vibrant red flowers. What's amazing about this plant is that the seed can lie dormant for decades. One bushfire, though, can 'burst' it awake and within no time it has germinated. Ah, the power of fire. Transformation.

Fire Warms
The primary reason for having an abundance of fire foods in our diet, apart from taste, is because they nourish us on a metabolic level by warming us. We are imbibing distilled sunlight. Not surprisingly, for many of us, the majority of our plant-based foods fall in the fire (fruit) category. Contrary to the opinion that we are, by nature, hunters, our body shows us that we are gatherers who are biologically designed to pluck, pick or dig our foods. Humans have little mouths compared to the size of their heads, and no claws or sharp teeth. Our body gives us all the proof we need of the food we are designed to eat.

Fire foods
Fruits, vegetables, seeds and nuts which grow above ground into a 'fruit' which can be plucked, such as peas, pumpkin, sweetcorn.

Fruits: Apple, orange, fig, grape, berry, avocado, banana, olive, etc.
Seeds: Chia, flax/linseed, pumpkin, quinoa, hemp, sunflower, sesame, etc.
Nuts: Coconut, almond, Brazil, hazel, macadamia, walnut, etc.
Grains: Rice, millet, amaranth, etc.
Legumes: Lentil, pea, bean, etc.

Earth and Root

While other little girls were playing with dolls, I was getting my hands and knees dirty playing Matchbox cars. They were driven on all the roads I'd created in the dirt. Mud pies were also a staple of my early years. You've probably guess it, but I wasn't a little girl in floaty pink dresses! Not to mention that I was expelled from ballet school, aged five, for not being able to touch my toes! Give me dirt any day.

It wasn't unusual for my siblings and I to cover our bodies in mud paint, or to swim naked in muddy dams. Even now, one of my favourite scents is petrichor: the smell of the earth when it rains. It truly ignites my senses, and makes me glad to be alive.

Earth is our foundation. We can see it, we can feel it. We talk about some people being 'down to earth'. These salt-of-the-earth souls are reliable and solid. You can depend on them no matter what. Unlike fire, water and air, earth is more stable. Those with planets in earth signs, are comforted by material security and substance, whether it is their own home, a vegetable garden, healthy bank account or a good massage.

We associate root vegetables primarily with Winter foods, and for good reason. They are grounding, and symbolic of survival. Energetically, they represent a 'going within'. Unlike the Yang energy of fire foods, earth ones are Yin. They represent the feminine deep and dark Earth.

Earth foods
Potato, sweet potato, carrot, parsnip, garlic, leeks, onion, fennel, black cumin, daikon, maca, jicama, black salsify, salsify, bush carrot, beetroot, rutabaga, burdock root, celeriac, parsley root, radish, turnip, ginger, pignut, cassava, Jerusalem artichoke, turmeric, etc.

A Zen blessing at mealtime:
"In this plate of food, I see the entire Universe supporting my existence."

Air and Flowers

Do you remember the old Mary Poppins' song *Let's Go Fly a Kite*? That was my first record, when I was about five years old.

As a child, I often had dreams of flying whereby I'd run down the hill behind our home, and miraculously I'd leave the ground and sail through the sky.

Despite a brewing cyclone, I flew a kite on my wedding day on the shores of Green Bay, Auckland, New Zealand. There's something about the air, the wind and the vast sky that captures the imagination. Even the most logical amongst us will surely have had moments of watching the clouds and wondering if they were making pictures.

I've always been enchanted by electrical storms, right from the earliest age. Even though we were warned by everyone around not to go outside during a storm, little minx that I was I'd sneak out and just stand there below the pewter skies as the shocking sparks of electric light sent forks in unpredictable directions. I felt empowered, and powerful, standing within the volatility of an electrical storm. It's one of the things I really miss about my native Australia. We look to the air sign, Aquarius, and its planetary ruler, Uranus, when assigning a placement for thunderstorms. Sudden. Quick. Shocking. Electrifying.

Air is the element that can't be seen or touched, and remains somewhat mysterious even though we get a strong sense of it from a thunderstorm or violent winds or even the hint of a gentle breeze. We crave fresh air when a room is stale. There is no predicting air, and although it is necessary to life, it eludes us in many ways. Astrologically, it rules the zodiac signs of Gemini, Libra and Aquarius.

Energetically, it has to do with abstract ideas, personal interaction, the gathering of information, workings of the mind, and perception.

Those people who have a strong 'air' influence in their birth chart tend to live in their mind. A bit like the kite in Mary Poppins reaching up to the atmosphere, these people's minds tend to live there, too. They're great at coming up with theories and solving problems.

Air foods
Any edible flower, for example: starflower (borage), viola, calendula, rose petals, etc.

Moon-infused water
If you don't feel inclined to eat flowers, there's another way to include the air element in your diet. While the Moon is transiting an air sign, place some spring water outside (in a glass jar), and then sip it throughout the day. This is particularly powerful at a Full or New Moon.

Water and Leaf

My earliest water-based memories are from just before we moved to live in the countryside. I was about five, and we lived in the outer suburbs of Brisbane, in Queensland, Australia. When a storm unleashed itself, the gutters would flood and send torrents of water along the edge of the street. I loved nothing better than to stand in there, and to feel the power of the water swoosh by my little legs.

Nearby was a place called Dead Horse Creek (no dead horses!), where my teenage sister, Heidi, would take me swimming.

Later, we moved to the countryside, and although we grew up in a drought-stricken place, water filled my days: we'd jump from the granite-based waterfall into the dam and swim amongst leeches. Other days, we'd ride bareback on our horses into the muddy manmade dams to seek out coolness from the scorching Australian sunshine.

Much of my childhood was enjoyed along the spring-fed creek. The pristine water, often sipped directly from our cupped hands, flowed down from high in the mountains.

My mother didn't take us to a doctor but instead chose to heal our ailments via holistic means. One such way was through the use of solarised coloured water. She would place a coloured glass of water in the sunlight all day, and the light would infuse it. Each colour represents a different energy useful in healing. For example, she would use blue to soothe our headaches, or red to help reduce shyness, and yellow to ease bedwetting.

During my pregnancy with my first daughter, I founded the National Waterbirth Trust in New Zealand as a way to help other mothers have access to information on birthing in water (the Internet was still in its infancy). My daughter was born gently and beautifully in a warm birthing pool in our bedroom.

Water has played a soothing role in my life, and even now one of my daily pleasures is a steaming hot shower. I love the sensation of being in a hot tub or a steam room, or my feet walking on wet grass. Whether we find refreshment walking alongside the tides of the ocean or sipping water from a stream or swimming in a pool, we can be sure that it will offer healing.

Energetically, water is to do with empathy, sensitivity and feelings. In psychological astrology, it represents our emotional self, and denotes intuition. One only has to think of great artesian basins (underground lakes) to understand how deep water seeps. If there's a hole or space, water will get in! Well, in terms of the energetics of water as a 'feeling' sign, the same thing happens. Those with strong water signs in their astrological chart will be highly empathetic, and may well be psychic, too. They are deeply attuned to the needs of others, and have a high emotional quotient.

Like the other elements, when water is uncontained it can cause devastation: floods, tsumanis, or ice and snow.

Water foods
Lettuce, endive, chicory, Oriental leaves, kale, rocket, lamb's lettuce, water and land cress, spinach, chard and beet leaves, pea sprouts, bean sprouts, asparagus, fennel leaves, celery, etc.

Herbs: basil, chives, dill, chervil, coriander, loveage, mint, parsley, salad burnet, sorrel, sweet Cecily, etc.

Leafy greens are mostly made of water, and are strongly affected by the Moon. As a gardener, if you're planting by the Moon, sow big leaves under the waxing Moon, and small leaves by the waning Moon.

How to thrive
on a wholefood diet

Make a choice to eat wholefoods
The easiest way to live a wholefood lifestyle is to ensure that any processed foods you buy have five ingredients or fewer. Avoid added sugar and refined grains. Quite simply, look for foods with the least processing.

Fruits and vegetables
Fill your basket or trolley primarily with fruits and vegetables. The best 'fast foods' you can eat are things like bananas, carrots, apples, grapes, nuts and seeds. They need no preparation, and can be thrown in your bag at a moment's notice. My husband insists that runner beans are a really fast food!

If you aim to ensure your diet consists of at least eighty-percent fresh fruits and vegetables, and then top up with healthy grains, legumes, seeds and nuts, you will find yourself thriving (assuming you also have plenty of sleep, sunshine, exercise, laughter and happy thoughts and feelings).

Plant-based protein
Nuts and seeds are nutrient dense, and contain healthy fats and proteins, minerals and vitamins. Try to eat a handful each day in their raw form. They can be eaten whole or ground up and sprinkled onto meals or in smoothies or home-made energy bars.

Complex carbohydrates

When choosing energy-giving carbs, look for things like quinoa, sweet potatoes, pumpkin and fruit rather than processed and sugary treats. Healthy carbs give you energy without making your blood-sugar levels plummet.

Sugar is not your friend

Oh yes, she may be sweet but she's the devil in disguise. Sugar is pretty much in everything that's processed. It's hard to avoid unless you make all your meals from scratch. Look for substitutes like dates, fresh fruit, pure maple syrup or coconut-blossom sugar. Commercial labeling has made different names for sugar, such as: sucrose, maltose, dextrose, fructose, glucose, galactose, lactose, high-fructose corn syrup, glucose solids, cane juice, dextrin, maltodextrin, dextran, barley malt, beet sugar, corn syrup, malt syrup, diatase, diatastic malt, fruit juice, fruit-juice concentrate, golden syrup, turbinado, sorghum syrup, etc.

Legumes and beans

If you think beans make you poop, fart, pass wind, bottom cough (or whatever word you want to use!), then I'll let you in on a little secret: This only happens if they haven't been soaked and rinsed properly. You can avoid this problem by cooking them yourself or rinsing those from a can super well! It's a shame to exclude them from your diet. They're nutritious and filling, and they help avoid blood-sugar fluctuations.

Become a planner

Rather than waiting till you're hungry to decide what to eat, think ahead! If you're clear about what meals to make for the next few days, you'll be better prepared when you shop. Write a menu, and stick to it.

Consciously plan your cooking time
If you've got time for TV or Facebook scrolling, then you've got time to make lovely meals for yourself and your family. It's a matter of prioritising your health and well-being. And if you feel you genuinely don't have time to create nourishing meals, then perhaps it's time to look at your overall lifestyle and see what needs to change. Perhaps you could find a few hours in the week to bulk cook some meals? If it feels out of reach, maybe you could ask yourself why your health isn't a number-one priority, and consider building your life around self-care.

Love-Kitchen Pantry

Having staples in your pantry, fruits in bowls, and root veg in baskets, and goodies in your fridge, will make your cooking life more enjoyable. Here are some suggestions:

Artichokes (marinated)
Gluten-free baking powder
Gluten-free bicarbonate of soda (baking soda)
Canned or dried beans: black, black-eyed, chilli, chickpeas, kidney, pinto, cannellini, haricot, etc.
Dried fruits: apricots, cranberries, Medjool dates, sultanas, raisins, etc.
Black olives
Green olives
Gluten-free breadcrumbs or ricecrumbs
Cold-pressed oils: sunflower, coconut, olive, avocado, macadamia
Cocoa powder
Coconut: milk, cream, sugar
Polenta (instant)
Cornflour
Quinoa
Flours:
Dove's Farm gluten-free self-raising flour
Dove's Farm gluten-free plain flour
Rice Flour
Chickpea flour (gram or besan)

Condiments

Condiments of the season, as my husband likes to say!

Garlic (fresh and dried)

Herbs: basil, bay leaves, chives, coriander (ground and berries), dill, Italian herbs, oregano, parsley, marjoram, mint, rosemary, thyme)

Tamari (wheat-free soya sauce)

Spices: cinnamon, cloves, chilli, five-spice, cumin seeds, ground cumin, curry, ginger, nutmeg, fennel seeds, cardamom

Smoked sea salt

Cornish sea salt

Himalayan pink salt

The four seasons are
salt, pepper, mustard and vinegar.

Maple syrup

Date syrup

Molasses (blackstrap)

Nuts: almonds, hazelnuts, peanuts, pecans, pine nuts, walnuts, Brazil nuts, cashews, etc.

Gluten-free porridge oats

Onions: white, red

Gluten-free spaghetti, pasta, lasagna

Organic crunchy peanut butter

Rice: organic brown basmati; Arborio, wild rice, split peas and lentils: red, Puy, green

Tofu: silky, firm

Tomato: passata (sieved tomatoes), tomato paste

Apple-cider vinegar

Organic vanilla paste

Marigold's vegan (gluten-free) bouillon powder

Balsamic vinegar

Xanthan gum
Nutritional Yeast Flakes *(gives a lovely cheesey flavour)*
Yeast Extract *(like Vegemite)*
Sun-dried tomatoes
Plant milk: almond, rice, cashew, coconut, soy, hazel

A Note on Ingredients
Salt
When I write salt, I'm not meaning table salt. Please don't use it. Ever. I primarily use Cornish sea salt, or Maldon sea salt, or Himalayan pink salt.

Pepper
I use coarse-ground black pepper, and my measurements are always based on that.

Coconut sugar
If I mention sugar, it will almost certainly be based on using coconut sugar as it is lower on the glycemic index (unless otherwise stated in the recipe). Coconut sugar is produced from the sap of cut flower buds of the coconut palm.

Transatlantic Translations
Coriander (cilantro), cornflour (maize starch), polenta (cornmeal)

Microwaves
I don't recommend microwaves because they destroy the 'essential energy' (enzymes) of a food.

Flax Eggs
Mix 1 tablespoon of flaxseeds or ground flaxseeds with 3 tablespoons of water and allow to sit for ten or so

minutes. This acts as an egg replacer.

Measurements
I use metric measurements
¼ cup = 60ml
1/3 cup = 80ml
½ cup = 125ml
1 cup = 250ml
¼ teaspoon = 1.25ml
½ teaspoon = 2.5ml
1 teaspoon = 5ml
2 teaspoons = 10ml
1 tablespoon = 20ml

Temperature Conversion

Gas	°F	°C	Fan
1	275	140	120
2	300	150	130
3	325	170	150
4	350	180	160
5	375	190	170
6	400	200	180
7	425	220	200
8	450	230	210
9	475	240	220

In my kitchen
For two decades, I cooked for a family of four. Old habits die hard! I'm adjusting to life as a family of two, now that our daughters are adults and not living at home. For the sake of habit, these recipes are designed to feed four, unless otherwise stated.

Love Notes

As a child, my evening meal almost always consisted mostly of raw vegetables: grated beetroot and carrot, sun-ripened tomatoes, alfalfa sprouts, slices of cucumber, succulent red peppers (capsicum in my native Australia), nut butter and more. Eating lots of raw vegetables was such a way of life, that it's never really left me, and most of the time my plate consists of anywhere between 50% and 80% salad.

My idea of salad is, quite simply, an abundance of leafy greens. This is different to what many restaurants now call salad, which can consist of cooked pasta and animal products.

However, I do enjoy a variety of salads, and I hope you enjoy this selection.

Salads

Black Bean and Corn Salad

5 cups cooked black beans, rinsed well
½ cup good-quality salad dressing (if you've got The Mystic
Cookfire, use the Mystic Salad dressing, page 370)
2 cups cooked corn kernels
1 red pepper, sliced thinly
1 green pepper, sliced thinly
1 yellow pepper, sliced thinly
3 spring onions, finely sliced
¼ cup fresh coriander leaves, finely chopped
1 teaspoon ground cumin
Juice of 1 lime
Salt and freshly ground pepper to taste

Combine all the ingredients in a serving bowl, and toss
well. Use the salad dressing to coat, but don't drown the
vegetables!

Blueberry Kale Salad

Two incredibly healthy foods join forces to have you bouncing off the ceiling with vibrant energy. I am so blessed to have several thriving blueberry bushes in my garden, and it is always my Autumnal joy to stand there, barefooted, plucking those delicious bursts of perfection, and storing them in my mouth for a few precious seconds. And baby-leaf kale is so easy to grow. Why not start a tub outside your door in a sunny spot?

5 cups baby-leaf kale
2 large handfuls blueberries
½ teaspoon sesame seeds

Lime and Sesame dressing:
Juice of 2 large limes
2 tablespoons tahini
1 tablespoon maple syrup
Pinch of sea salt

Mix the dressing ingredients until smooth, then mix well through the kale leaves, and use your hands to massage it into the leaves to soften. Add the berries and seeds. Note: if you can't get baby-leaf kale, use mature kale but massage the leaves for longer (and make sure to remove chunky stems).

Beetroot Tabbouleh Salad

Tabbouleh comes from the Arabic *tabulah*, and is a vegetarian salad traditionally made of tomatoes, parsley, mint, bulgar wheat, onion, and seasoned with olive oil, lemon juice and salt. It's delicious and substantial. This is a gluten-free take on it, with a pink twist! Enjoy!

1 cup wild rice (soaked for two to three days), and rinsed each day (do make sure the rice isn't old, or it won't sprout)
2 large beetroots
½ cup sunflower seeds, soaked overnight
¼ cup sesame seeds, lightly toasted in a dry pan
1 cup ripe tomatoes, chopped
Handful fresh parsley, finely chopped
Handful mint leaves, finely chopped
Three spring onions, finely chopped

Ginger Dressing
2 tablespoons good-quality olive oil
1 tablespoon apple-cider vinegar
Juice of one lemon
1 teaspoon maple syrup
1 tablespoon finely grated ginger
Pinch of salt

The rice will have split open when it has been soaked for long enough. Once sprouted, rinsed and drained, place in a glass bowl, and cover with about half of the dressing.

Grate the beetroot, and mix into the rice. Add the rest of the ingredients, and the other half of the dressing. Mix well.

Roasted Fennel Salad

I'm fussy about the olive oil I use, and always go for the finest quality I can find. I was recently introduced to something that leaves everything I've ever used far behind. My friend Cassandra, and her husband, Peter, press oil from olives at their home in Portugal. I absolutely LOVE using this oil (and because it's so damn gorgeous I use it ridiculously liberally!), and the aroma when I open the jar makes me swoon like a lovesick fool. It's like a perfectly delicious smoked olive. Well, that's the best description I can come up with. Heavenly. When I ran out, and found myself standing in front of the large collection of olive oils in my supermarket, I could almost feel myself pouting, and my inner voice saying "But I want their Portuguese olive oil!"

1 fennel bulb per person, sliced in 3cm sections
A couple of oranges (or grapefruit), peeled, and thinly sliced
3 tablespoons white balsamic vinegar
3 tablespoons olive oil
Pinch of sea salt
1 spring onion, chopped
1 bunch fresh mint, thinly sliced

Preheat the oven to 190C. Roast the fennel with olive oil, balsamic vinegar and salt, and cook for about 20 minutes. Place on a plate with the oranges, and sprinkle over the spring onion and mint.

Almond and Broccoli Salad

2 cups cooked quinoa
1 cup raw almonds
2 tablespoons sunflower seeds
4 teaspoons sesame seeds
4 tablespoons olive oil
6 tablespoons lemon juice
4 cups broccoli florets
1 cup baby-leaf spinach
Sea salt

Steam the broccoli for five minutes. Meanwhile, in a processor, add almonds and seeds, and mix for about ten seconds. Combine all the ingredients in a bowl, and mix well.

Chicory and Raspberry Salad

This is one of my favourite salads. It's a fabulous mix of bitter and sweet. I guess it is life summed up in a mouthful of food!

1 cup raspberries
3 heads chicory
3 tablespoons olive oil
1 tablespoon balsamic vinegar
1 tablespoon maple syrup
Pinch of salt and black pepper

Slice the chicory lengthwise, and cook for about five minutes in a pan with the seasonings. When tender, place on a plate and mix through the raspberries.

When you realize how perfect everything is,
you will tilt your head back and laugh at the sky.
Buddha

Watercress and Fennel Salad

Watercress, like pumpkin seeds, should be a staple in any reproductive man's life. Rich in zinc, it's a superfood which tends not to get much press.

2 handfuls watercress
3 fennel bulbs, finely sliced
3 tablespoons olive oil
Pinch of salt
Freshly ground coarse black pepper
Juice and zest of 2 limes
150g vegan feta cheese or smoked tofu, crumbled

Whisk the lime juice, zest, salt, pepper and olive oil, then add the fennel and marinade for twenty minutes. When ready to serve, place the watercress on plates. Put the fennel on top, then add the feta or tofu.

Tom's Big-Ass Salad

I once shared a photo on social media of a large salad I had eaten in a Glaswegian café, and simply titled it: "big-ass salad". My friend Tom said that if my next recipe book had a salad by that name, he'd buy the book! Here it is, Tom Blackwell.

Just to be clear, it's the salad that has the big ass, not Tom! In fact, he tells me his is quite petite!

Per person
1 handful dark leafy greens, such as rocket, mizuna, spinach, and baby-leaf kale
½ cup cucumber slices (thin)
½ cup carrot sticks (thin)
½ cup baby corn, cut in half lengthwise
2 spring onions, finely chopped
½ avocado, peeled and sliced
¼ cup alfalfa sprouts
¼ cup sunflower seeds, lightly toasted
Splash of tamari (drizzle on seeds when they're toasted)

Arrange the vegetable ingredients into a wide shallow bowl or plate, then sprinkle with tamari-infused sunflower seeds.

Drizzle with the Mystic Dressing (recipe in my book The Mystic Cookfire) or dressing of your choice. Enjoy! And, get this, you won't end up with a big ass!

Coriander and Chickpea Salad

2 cans chickpeas, rinsed and drained
2 ripe tomatoes, chopped
½ red onion, finely chopped
Handful of fresh coriander, chopped
Drizzle of olive oil
1 tablespoon lime juice
Pinch of cumin
Pinch of chipotle chilli
Pinch of salt

Blend oil, juice and seasonings, then the chickpeas, vegetables and coriander. Mix well.

Don't dig your grave with your own knife and fork.
English Proverb

Mint and Mango Salad

1 can black beans, rinsed, drained
1 cup cooked quinoa, rinsed, drained
1 fresh mango, cubed
1 cucumber, seeds removed, diced
1 cup mint, chopped
6 tablespoons olive oil
2 tablespoons lime juice
1 tablespoon maple syrup
1 clove garlic, finely chopped
Salt and pepper

Whisk the olive oil, lime juice, and garlic. Add the rest of the ingredients and mix well, then chill the salad for an hour.

Spicy Cumin and Coconut Cauliflower Salad

Coconut oil for frying
4 cups cauliflower florets
1 cup butterbeans, drained and rinsed
4 cups baby-kale leaves
1 tablespoon lime juice
Pinch cumin seeds
Salt
Pepper

On low to medium heat, sauté the cauliflower in coconut oil until brown, then add the cumin seeds. After a few minutes, add the kale, butterbeans, lime juice, and season with salt and pepper to taste.

The act of putting into your mouth
what the earth has grown
is perhaps your most
direct interaction with the earth.
Frances Moore Lappé

Spinach and Chickpea Salad
with Lime Dressing

Chickpeas
6 cups cooked chickpeas
250g baby spinach leaves
2 cups coriander, chopped
½ cup red onion, chopped

Lime dressing
¼ cup lime juice
2 tablespoons olive oil
2 cloves garlic, finely chopped
1 teaspoon ground cumin
2 teaspoons maple syrup
Pinch of salt
Pinch of pepper

Rinse and drain the chickpeas. Place spinach and coriander in a food processor and chop well, then place in a bowl with the chopped onion, and chickpeas. Mix well.

Whisk together the dressing ingredients, and pour over the chickpea mix. You can leave it overnight.

Love Notes

Soups

It's fair to say that there's a handsome collection of soups in my first recipe book, The Mystic Cookfire.

As far as hot foods go, I could live off soup. It's warm, nourishing and so easy to put together. Nothing says "home sweet home" more than soup simmering on the stovetop on a bitterly cold Winter's day. Indeed, when I once asked my daughter what she thought of when she heard the word "home", she replied: "soup simmering on the stove".

Worries go better with soup than without.
Yiddish proverb

Ginger and Coconut Lentil Soup

Coconut oil
1 onion, chopped
2 cloves garlic, chopped
2 tablespoons fresh ginger, finely grated
2 tablespoons tomato paste
2 tablespoons curry powder
½ teaspoon cayenne pepper
4 cups vegetable bouillon
500ml coconut cream
2 cups red lentils
4 cups baby-leaf spinach
Salt and pepper

Sauté the onion, garlic and ginger in coconut oil for a few minutes, then add the tomato paste, curry and cayenne. Mix well, then add the bouillon, cream and lentils. Simmer on low heat for at least half an hour, or until the lentils are soft, then season with salt and pepper according to taste. Add the spinach, and allow to wilt.

Hungarian Dill and Mushroom Soup

Olive oil
2 onions, chopped
2 cloves garlic, chopped
1kg mixed mushrooms (wild, button, shiitake, etc)
¼ cup tamari
2 teaspoons dried dill
2 teaspoons smoked paprika
Pinch of black pepper
Squeeze of lemon juice
¼ cup plain flour
4 cups vegetable bouillon
2 cups unsweetened plant milk

Sauté onions in a little olive oil (or water) for a few minutes, then add the garlic and mushrooms, and cook until they sweat. Add seasonings, then cook until there is a fair bit of liquid from the mushroom sweat. Add the flour, and mix well. Slowly add the bouillon, then the milk. Simmer for about 20 minutes on low heat. Note: if preferred, you can use coconut (or other plant-based) cream instead of milk.

Roast Garlic and Cherry Tomato Soup

I'm one of the middle children of eight kids. As someone who loved one-on-one time with my mum, about the only way I could secure such quality time was to engineer sick days from school. Truth is, Mum always knew I wasn't sick (I was a robust little creature!) and she would let me take days off school from time to time anyway. I detested school, so it was an added joy to be at home with my mum. She often made us tomato soup garnished with fresh parsley, and served with peanut butter on rye crackers. We'd dine outside in the garden under the beautiful warm Australian sunshine. Needless to say, tomato soup only has positive memories for me.

4 cups cherry tomatoes
6 cloves garlic, peeled
2 onions, sliced into wedges
3 cups vegetable bouillon
Olive oil
Salt
Pepper
1 cup fresh basil leaves

Heat the oven to 220C. The exquisite taste of this soup relies on slow roasting the vegetables: Place them on a baking tray, and drizzle with olive oil. Bake for about 25 minutes, then place vegetables and liquid into a soup pan. Add the bouillon and simmer for fifteen minutes. Blend the soup, in whole or part, and adjust taste with salt and pepper, Stir through ripped basil leaves just before serving.

Thyme and Cauliflower Soup

Olive oil
1 onion, chopped
1 clove garlic, chopped
3 cups vegetable bouillon
1 large cauliflower
3 potatoes, chopped
1 teaspoon fresh thyme, chopped
Salt and pepper, to taste

Sauté the onion and garlic in oil for a few minutes, then add the bouillon and potatoes. Bring to the boil, then simmer for 20 minutes. Add the cauliflower and thyme. Cover the pot, and cook for a few more minutes. Blend the soup, then adjust taste by adding salt and pepper to suit.

Red Pepper Soup
with Maple and Balsamic Reduction

Olive oil
1 red onion, chopped
1 sweet potato, peeled and chopped
1 teaspoon ground cumin
¼ teaspoon red-pepper flakes
1 clove garlic, chopped
6 cups vegetable bouillon
4 large red peppers, chopped

Balsamic Reduction
1 cup balsamic vinegar
¼ cup maple syrup

Sauté the red onion and sweet potato for several minutes, then add the garlic and seasonings. Sauté for a few minutes, then add the bouillon and peppers. Simmer for about half an hour. Blend. Season with salt and pepper.

Bring the vinegar and maple syrup to the boil then simmer for about twenty minutes until thickened. Allow to cool. Once the soup is in bowls, drizzle with the balsamic.

White Bean and Spinach Soup

Spinach is an edible flowering plant native to central and western Asia. It's an excellent source of vitamin K, vitamin A, manganese, folate, magnesium, iron, copper, vitamin B2, vitamin B6, vitamin E, calcium, potassium, vitamin C, phosphorus, vitamin B1, zinc, protein, and choline.

Olive oil
1 onion, finely chopped
8 carrots, sliced
2 cloves garlic, chopped
2 tablespoons vegetable bouillon powder
1 can chopped tomatoes
2 teaspoons good-quality curry powder
Pinch of cinnamon
Pinch of ground nutmeg
500g cooked white beans, drained and rinsed
2 generous handfuls of baby spinach leaves, well rinsed
Salt and freshly ground pepper to taste

Sauté the onion, carrot and garlic in oil (or water) for about five minutes. Add a litre of water, bouillon powder, tomatoes, beans and seasonings. Simmer for twenty minutes. Add the spinach, and cook until wilted. Check the seasonings, and add more salt and pepper, and water, if desired.

Curried Aubergine Soup

Aubergines might not be the first vegetable you think of when planning to cook soup, but don't skip by this recipe. Aubergines are absolute treasure troves at soaking up flavours. They're a good source of vitamins B1, B6 and potassium, and high in copper, magnesium and manganese.

Olive oil
1 large onion, finely chopped
4 cloves garlic, finely chopped
3 celery stalks, finely chopped
1 tablespoon plain flour
2 large sweet potatoes, peeled and finely chopped
2 large aubergines, peeled and finely chopped
2 teaspoons curry powder
2 tablespoons maple syrup or coconut sugar
3 cups coconut cream
Pinch or two of salt
Freshly ground black pepper
¼ cup fresh parsley, finely chopped

Sauté the onion, celery and garlic until translucent. Keep moist by adding more oil or water if necessary. Mix in the flour and stir through. Add the sweet potato, aubergine, curry powder and water (just enough to cover the vegetables). Simmer until the potatoes are tender, then add the coconut cream and sweetener. Add salt and pepper, and simmer for a few more minutes. Garnish with parsley.

Creamy Fresh Thyme and Tomato Soup

800g canned tomatoes, chopped
1 cup coconut or rice milk
1 onion, chopped
4 cloves garlic, chopped
1tablespoon vegetable bouillon powder
Pinch of salt
Pinch or two of coarse-ground black pepper
1 tablespoon fresh thyme leaves
1 cup water
Olive oil

Sauté onion and garlic in oil or water for a few minutes, then add the remaining ingredients, and cook gently for about 10 – 15 minutes. Blend, in whole or part, if desired.

Curried Coconut and Lentil Soup

1kg butternut squash, peeled, and cut into cubes
1 onion, chopped
3 cloves garlic, chopped
Chunk of fresh ginger root, peeled and chopped
1 cup red lentils
4 cups vegetable bouillon
¼ teaspoon smoked paprika
1 tablespoon cumin seeds
1 tablespoon black mustard seeds
250ml coconut milk
250ml coconut cream
Pinch of salt
Handful fresh coriander leaves, chopped
Coconut oil

Sauté the mustard seeds and cumin seeds for a minute or two, then add the onion, garlic and ginger. Continue cooking until the onion softens, then add the lentils and squash. Stir, then add bouillon and simmer. Cook gently for twenty minutes until the squash is tender. Add salt and pepper to taste, and coconut milk and cream, then top with the coriander when serving.

Curried Cauliflower and Chickpea Soup

This delightful African-style soup is rich with spices, peanut butter, and is also a great source of protein with the chickpeas.

Olive or coconut oil
1 large onion, peeled and chopped
½ teaspoon cumin seeds
1 tablespoon finely grated ginger root
1 small jalapeño, seeded and finely chopped
3 cloves garlic, chopped
4 cups vegetable bouillon
½kg sweet potatoes, peeled and cut into cubes
1 tablespoon curry powder, divided in half
Pinch of cinnamon
1 large cauliflower, broken into florets
2 cups cooked chickpeas
500g can tomatoes, chopped
2-4 cups water
Pinch of salt
Pinch of cayenne pepper
2 tablespoons crunchy peanut butter

Sauté the onion in oil or water for a few minutes, then add the cumin seeds, ginger, garlic, jalapeño, and cook for half a minute, stirring the whole time. Add the sweet potatoes, bouillon, half of the curry powder, and cinnamon. Bring to a boil, then simmer for about half an hour till the potato has softened. Then, add the cauliflower, chickpeas, and tomatoes to the pan. Cover the cauliflower in water. Add the rest of the curry, salt, and cayenne. Cook for twenty minutes, then add the peanut butter and mix well.

Spiced Tomato and Kale Soup

I come from a line of German ancestors and ancestresses. One of my aunties can't understand all the fuss about kale being a superfood. She said that when they were growing up, it was a staple of their diet.

2 handfuls kale, thinly sliced (unless using baby-leaf kale)
Coconut or olive oil
2 garlic cloves, finely chopped
1 onion, chopped
2 red peppers
2 bay leaves
Pinch of ground cumin
1 teaspoon cayenne pepper
Pinch of ground coriander
Pinch of smoked paprika
400g can tomatoes, chopped
6 cups vegetable bouillon
1 cup red lentils, rinsed
Salt
Pepper

Sauté the onion and garlic in oil for several minutes, then add the peppers. After a few more minutes, add the bay leaves and the spices, tomatoes, bouillon and lentils. Cook for half an hour at a simmer, then when the lentils are cooked, add the kale. Once the leaves have wilted, adjust seasonings if desired.

Sweet and Sour Summer Corn Chowder

As a barefoot child growing up in rural Australia, I have many happy memories of playing hide and seek with my siblings in the neighbour's corn fields. I love to eat corn fresh off the cob. If you prefer yours cooked, why not try this exotic soup?

5 cups corn kernels
2 cans coconut milk
1 red onion, chopped
3 cloves garlic, chopped
1 inch fresh ginger, finely grated
1 tablespoon turmeric
2 tablespoons nutritional yeast
Juice of two limes
3 cups water
Pinch of salt
1 tablespoon maple syrup
Pinch of black pepper

Sauté onion, garlic and ginger for a few minutes, then add corn, coconut milk, water, salt, pepper and maple. Simmer uncovered for half an hour, then add the remaining ingredients and stir well.

Coriander and Cumin-infused Lentil Soup

Cumin is one of those spices that brings out the red-blooded woman in me. It's reminiscent of the smell of a healthy man. I used to think that perhaps it was just me, and *my* man, but many of my female friends say the erotic aroma of cumin has the same effect on them.

2 cups Puy lentils, uncooked
8 cups vegetable bouillon
1 large onion, chopped
2 cloves garlic, chopped
2 large carrots, sliced
1 celery stick, chopped
2 sweet potatoes, cut into large cubes
2 bay leaves
1 teaspoon ground coriander
Pinch of ground cumin
Freshly ground pepper, to taste
Salt
Two large handfuls fresh baby-leaf spinach
2 teaspoons lemon juice

Cook the lentils until tender, rinse well, then return to the soup pan. Add all the ingredients (except spinach), and cook until the sweet potatoes are tender. Remove the bay leaves, and add spinach and lemon juice.

Moroccan Lentil and Lemon Soup

My sister Heidi is amazing. She turned an empty building into an incredible Moroccan restaurant on Queensland's Airlie Beach. Filled with lush plants, mirrors, colourful cushions, and Moroccan lanterns, the décor was a perfect match for her imaginative and interesting cooking.

Olive oil
2 large onions, finely chopped
3 celery stalks, finely chopped
3 cloves garlic, finely chopped
6 cups water
1 cup dried Puy lentils, rinsed
1 teaspoon turmeric
1 teaspoon cumin
1 teaspoon grated fresh ginger root
1 teaspoon cinnamon
2 cups diced ripe tomatoes
2 cans chickpeas, drained and rinsed
Juice of a lemon
Fresh zest of half a lemon
½ cup chopped fresh coriander
Salt

Sauté the onions in olive oil until clear. Add the celery and garlic, and sauté for another five minutes. Add the water, lentils and spices. Simmer for thirty minutes, then add tomatoes and chickpeas. Adjust with more water and spices if necessary. Over low heat, cook for another fifteen minutes. Add coriander and lemon juice. Add salt to taste.

Love Notes

Casseroles, bakes, roasts, lasagne and stews

Black Bean and Yellow Pepper Masala

The aromatic spices in this dish conjure up the cuisine of Northern India. The name of this spice is derived from the Hindi language. This hot spice has many variations depending on the geographical location. Indeed, each generation and family have their own traditional garam masala recipe.

Garam means 'heat', and according to the ancient healing modality of the Ayurvedic, it warms the body. What this means is that it lights the digestive fire, otherwise known as *agni*. To keep it working optimally, it needs a specific type of warmth.

Garam masala raises the body temperature, which increases metabolism. Without this digestive warmth, bodily toxins build up as a result of a sluggish metabolism.

Olive oil
1 large onion, chopped
2 to 3 cloves garlic, chopped
3 cups cooked black beans, well rinsed
3 yellow peppers, diced
1 chilli, finely chopped
2 teaspoons garam masala
½ teaspoon turmeric
1 teaspoon ground cumin
2 teaspoons grated fresh ginger
2 large ripe tomatoes, chopped
1 tablespoon lemon juice, or more, to taste
¼ cup finely chopped fresh coriander
Salt to taste

Sauté the onion until translucent, then add the garlic. After a few minutes, add the beans, chilli, seasonings, tomatoes, lemon juice, and about a quarter of a cup water. Simmer, then cook over low heat for 10 minutes. Be sure to stir. Stir in the coriander, and add salt to taste. Serve with basmati rice, quinoa or poppadoms.

The more you eat, the less flavour;
the less you eat, the more flavour.
Chinese Proverb

Red Lentil and Brazil Nut Loaf

I chose to go completely gluten-free a couple of years ago when discovering I had low thyroid. Gluten, along with chlorine, is detrimental to optimal thyroid health.

In my twenties, I lived in New Zealand for eight years. The country is known for having low selenium levels in the soil. Selenium is an essential mineral for the thyroid, and so I ensure that I eat a handful of raw Brazil nuts each day as they're one of the richest sources of this mineral.

Olive oil
1 cup red lentils
2.5 cups vegetable bouillon
1 bay leaf
1 leek, finely chopped
1 red pepper, chopped
1 cup mushrooms, chopped
1 cup grated carrot
1 cup Brazil nuts, chopped
1 garlic clove, chopped
1 tablespoon lemon juice
1 tablespoon tomato paste
1 tablespoon smoked paprika
3 tablespoons nutritional yeast flakes
2 cups bread crumbs or rice crumbs
2 tablespoons fresh parsley, chopped

Sauce
1 tablespoon tomato paste
1 teaspoon smoked paprika
1 can crushed tomatoes

¼ cup vegetable bouillon
1 teaspoon dried sage
1 tablespoon maple syrup

Preheat the oven to 190C. Line the loaf pan with parchment paper.

Cook the lentils with the bay leaf and bouillon, and simmer for twenty minutes. Remove the bay leaf. Sauté the onion, leek, red pepper, mushrooms, and carrot. After a few minutes, add the remaining ingredients. Ensure they're all mixed well, then press into your loaf tin. Bake, covered, for thirty minutes. Uncover, and bake for another thirty minutes.

Sauce: To make the sauce, simmer all ingredients for twenty minutes. Pour over the loaf when serving.

Creamy Kale Bake

This is one of those 'quick and easy' dishes, and yet it's just so nourishing.

1 butternut squash, peeled, and cut into cubes
½ kilo potatoes (white or sweet), peeled, and cut into cubes
8 large kale leaves or 4 cups of baby-leaf kale
2 cups coconut cream
½ cup milk
2 teaspoons vegetable bouillon powder
Salt and pepper, to taste
Vegan cheese

Preheat oven to 185C. Remove the stalks from the kale, and cut the leaves thinly. Place the vegetables into a casserole dish, and mix. In another bowl, mix the cream, milk, seasonings, and then pour over the vegetables. Ensure the liquid is evenly distributed. Bake for about 20 to 25 minutes (stirring, if needed); then, if desired, sprinkle with grated cheese a few minutes before the end of cooking time.

Spinach and Polenta Bakes

There's something about well-made polenta that epitomises the best of comfort food! Though, you do need to be mindful of the right brand. I've come across one that resembled sawdust! Not good. I use my supermarket's own brand, and it comes out perfectly every time.

500g polenta
Olive oil or coconut oil
2 to 3 cloves garlic, finely chopped
Two cans black beans, drained and rinsed
1 red pepper, chopped
1 teaspoon ground cumin
300g fresh baby spinach
Salt and freshly ground pepper to taste

Prepare the polenta as per packet instructions. Once cooked, allow to cool and thicken some more. In an egg ring, or simply putting scoops onto baking paper, set out circles of polenta. When they have set, grill until they are golden.

Sauté the garlic over a low heat for a couple of minutes, then add the beans, pepper, and cumin. Cook over medium heat for several minutes, then add the spinach so that it wilts. Season, then remove from the heat.

Spoon the spinach mixture onto three polenta circles for each person. This can be served with a salad if it is a main meal, or on its own as a snack or starter.

Rosemary-infused Chickpeas

Chickpeas, also known as garbanzo beans, actually look like little chicken heads. Creepy, really, but my, oh my, are they nutritious! They're also really versatile and can be used for all manner of things, whether it is whole in a stew, or ground into flour (gram or besan) and used for pancakes and farinatas. You can even use the liquid from a tin of chickpeas to make an egg-free pavlova! This is a simple, yet delicious, recipe with lots of oomph!

4 cups cooked chickpeas
2 red onions, finely chopped
3 cloves garlic, chopped
2 cups chopped tomatoes
½ cup red pepper, chopped
2 tablespoons apple-cider vinegar
Olive oil
1 tablespoon freshly grated ginger
2 teaspoons maple syrup
2 teaspoons mustard seeds
1 teaspoon dried oregano
1 teaspoon dried rosemary
1 teaspoon sea salt
Freshly ground black pepper
2 dried bay leaves

Preheat the oven to 200°C. Combine all the ingredients in a baking dish, except the bay leaves. When mixed well, add the leaves. Bake for half an hour. Remove from the oven, and stir. Bake for another 45 minutes. When serving, remove the bay leaves. Serve with rice or quinoa.

Tomato and Ginger Chickpeas

I swear that sometimes the quickest and simplest meals to prepare are often the tastiest. This is a fab example. Now, it could just be because I absolutely love ginger, but the combination of spices is divine.

Olive oil
1 large onion, sliced
4 cups tomatoes, chopped
2 tablespoons grated fresh ginger root
3 cups cooked chickpeas
1 teaspoon cumin
1 teaspoon cinnamon
¼ teaspoon turmeric
Salt and freshly ground pepper to taste
Handful fresh coriander, chopped

Sauté the onions, ginger, and tomatoes until the tomatoes are soft, then add the remaining ingredients and simmer for fifteen minutes. Serve on a bed of mashed sweet potatoes, alongside your favourite salad.

Curry-Roasted Cauliflower

1 head cauliflower, cut into florets
2 cups cooked chickpeas
3 tablespoons olive oil
2 garlic cloves, chopped
1 teaspoon ground turmeric
1 teaspoon ground cumin
1 teaspoon ground coriander
Pinch of salt
Handful of fresh coriander, chopped

Preheat the oven to 205C.

Mix all the ingredients, then place into a casserole dish and roast for about half an hour to forty minutes, turning once or twice in that time. Serve with quinoa and salad.

Courgette and Pineapple Chilli

If it's a good growing season, then it's inevitable that you'll end up with a glut of courgettes. Here's a great way to use up a bunch. Enjoy the dance of sweet pineapple and spicy chilli on your tongue. It's amazing!

1 large onion, chopped
1 large red pepper, chopped
4 cloves garlic, chopped
1 chilli, finely chopped
1 can chopped tomatoes
2 cans black beans, rinsed and drained
2 cups vegetable bouillon
1 tablespoon smoked paprika
1 teaspoon ground cumin
2 teaspoons dried oregano
Pinch of black pepper
1 teaspoon salt
3 courgettes, cut into small cubes
1 cup crushed pineapple and juice

Sauté the onion in olive oil, and cook until golden. Add the pepper and chilli, and cook until softened. Add the garlic, tomatoes, beans, bouillon, and seasonings (not courgettes and pineapple). Bring to a boil, then reduce heat and simmer for 15 minutes. Add the courgettes and pineapple, and simmer until tender. Check seasonings, adding more to taste, and serve with rice, quinoa or pasta.

Lentil Walnut Bolognese

Bolognese originates from the Italian city of Bologna, and is founded on a simple mix of meat, onions and tomatoes. There's no meat here, but we keep the rich tradition of onion and colourful tomatoes, and create a meaty texture from those beloved earthy foods: walnuts and lentils. You can serve this with spaghetti or atop baked potatoes, on rice or quinoa, or even on sandwiches.

1 cup onion, chopped
3 cloves garlic, chopped
1 can chopped tomatoes
1 tube tomato paste (200g)
3 cups water
1.5 cups green lentils (ideally soaked overnight, then rinsed well)
1.5 tablespoons maple syrup or coconut sugar
1 cup chopped walnuts
2 tablespoons oregano (fresh or dried)
Olive oil
1 teaspoon salt
Coarse-ground black pepper

Heat the onion and garlic in a little olive oil. When translucent, add the tomatoes, water, lentils, and sweetener, and stir well. Cover the pot, and simmer for at least half an hour.

When the lentils are cooked (soft, but still in shape), add the tomato paste, walnuts, salt, pepper, and oregano and mix well.

Black Bean and Courgette Casserole

Black beans are such a nutritious food that it's worth serving them up several times a week in one form or another. This simple recipe will fill the emptiest tummy. The beauty of beans is that they release their energy slowly, keeping you active for longer. Serve with brown rice, corn chips and cheese, or on a baked sweet potato.

Olive oil
1 cup onion, chopped
1 red pepper, chopped
2 cups cooked black beans, rinsed and drained
2 courgettes, sliced
1 cup tomato, chopped
1 small chilli, finely chopped
2 teaspoons smoked paprika
1 teaspoon dried oregano
½ teaspoon ground cumin
Salt and pepper, to taste

Preheat the oven to 200° C. Sauté the onion until clear, then add the pepper. When softened, add the remaining ingredients and cook until tender.

Butternut and Aduki Bean Hotpot

What is it about aduki beans? They're so quick to cook, and nourishing to boot. I love that they're jam-packed with lots of nutrients, and at the same time make a rather awesome comfort food. Now, don't be like my friend Christine and forget to cook the beans first! Because, clever as I am, I can't come and magic them into "cookedness" once you've added all the other ingredients!

Olive oil
2 onions, chopped
4 cloves garlic, chopped
5 cups cooked aduki beans (cook them first, Christine)
1 cup butternut, peeled, then cut into 1cm cubes
1 carrot, sliced
3 peppers, chopped
Generous pinches of sea salt
Generous grindings of coarse black pepper
3 tablespoons maple syrup
3 tablespoons bouillon powder
200g tomato paste
Water

Topping:
5 medium potatoes (white or sweet), thinly sliced, for placing on top of beans.

Preheat oven to 200C. Sauté onions for a few minutes, then add the garlic. Cook for a few minutes, then add the remaining vegetables and sauté until soft. Add the cooked beans and seasonings. Add the tomato paste and water. Allow to cook for ten minutes. Adjust the seasonings to suit. Place in a casserole dish, and arrange the sliced potatoes on top (the potatoes will need to be sliced thinly, and can also be steamed briefly, first, to speed up baking time). Drizzle liberally with olive oil, and then sprinkle with coarse-ground black pepper and sea salt. If you have sesame seeds, they're lovely sprinkled on top, too. Bake for about half an hour, until potatoes are soft and golden.

Lemon and Ginger Quinoa

It's handy to have a large bowl of cooked quinoa in the fridge just waiting to be used for a sweet or savoury dish. This meal makes a quick, tasty and nutritious lunch. Serve with salad or inside Romaine lettuce leaves.

3 cups cooked quinoa, cooled
1 carrot, julienned
1 yellow pepper, sliced
1 onion, chopped
3 cloves garlic, chopped
2 cups baby spinach leaves
2 spring onions, sliced
Handful green beans, chopped
½ cup butternut pumpkin, chopped
1 inch ginger root, finely grated
1 organic lemon zest, finely grated
1 teaspoon smoked paprika
Sea salt (generous pinches)
Freshly ground coarse black pepper
Olive oil

Sauté the onion, garlic, spring onions and pepper in olive oil (or water). Add the remaining vegetables and seasonings, and cook until the butternut is tender. When cooked, mix well, then add quinoa. Ensure the flavourings are well distributed.

Mushroom and Thyme Risotto

Mushrooms. I sure do love them! I could eat mushrooms every day, and often do. I never tire of them. They're fungi, and have their own place in the plant kingdom. They're naturally gluten-free, and offer important nutrients, such as selenium, B vitamins, Vitamin D, potassium and so much more. I particularly enjoy them because they have a filling texture, and really add substance to any meal.

3 cups cooked quinoa
2-3 cups mixed mushrooms, such as button, shiitake, wild, chestnut
1 red onion
8 cloves garlic
1 tablespoon fresh thyme leaves
2 teaspoons sea salt
Freshly ground black pepper
Olive oil
1½ cups vegetable bouillon or white wine

Sauté the onion and garlic until soft, then add the mushrooms and cook until soft; then season to taste. Add the drained quinoa to the pan, and add a quarter of the wine (or bouillon, if preferred). When the wine has evaporated, add the remaining wine. Simmer. Serve with a seasonal salad.

Orange and Maple Marinated Tofu

Ever so quick to prepare, and beautiful to eat, I love the lightness of this dish, and the zing of the different flavours.

Two blocks of tofu (drain both sides on a kitchen paper towel)

Mix the following ingredients together:
2 oranges, sliced
1 orange, juiced
1 cup maple syrup
Inch of grated ginger root
Pinches of sea salt
Generous pinch of ground black pepper

Preheat oven to 150C.

In an ideal world, you would marinate the tofu overnight. In a busy world, you might have about 15 minutes to let the ingredients sit. The longer you can leave it, the better. Pour half the marinade into a casserole dish.

Slice each block of tofu in half sideways, then in half from the top, and lay in a casserole dish. Pour the remaining marinade over the top, and bake for 40 minutes. Serve with seasonal steamed vegetables.

Spinach and Nutmeg Quinoa Bake

A superbly light dish that somehow falls into the category of comfort food! This is a family favourite.

4 cups cooked quinoa, or two cups uncooked
2 tablespoons vegetable bouillon powder (to put in the quinoa cooking water)
Olive oil, sunflower or coconut oil
1 cup coconut yoghurt
2 onions (one red, if desired), chopped
5 cloves garlic, chopped
2 teaspoons nutmeg
Pinch of cayenne pepper
4 cups baby spinach leaves
3 cups coconut cream
2 teaspoons organic lemon zest
¼ teaspoon freshly ground black pepper
1 grated carrot
1 teaspoon turmeric
1 teaspoon egg replacer/flax egg

Cook the quinoa in water and bouillon, until the 'tail' comes out of the seed.

Preheat the oven to 175C. Oil a 20x20cm baking dish or line with baking paper.

Sauté the chopped onions and garlic in a little oil for several minutes, until clear.

Add the nutmeg and cayenne, then the spinach, and sauté for a few minutes. Combine with the yoghurt, quinoa, egg replacer, carrot, lemon zest, pepper, turmeric and cream. When well mixed, pour into the baking dish. Bake for one hour or until the edges are brown. After cooking, leave to set for ten minutes. Can be served hot or cold. Perfect for lunch boxes.

Serves six as a main dish. Serve with steamed greens or salad.

Baked Lentils with Pear, Sweet Potato and Maple

Everything about this dish says: Autumn. It's a vibrant mix of earthy with a hint of sweet. Be warned: it's moreish.

4 cups Puy lentils, cooked
2 onions, chopped
5 garlic cloves, chopped
2 pears, cored and chopped
1 sweet potato, chopped into 1cm cubes
4 tomatoes, chopped
3 tablespoons maple syrup
1½ teaspoons salt
Generous pinch of coarse-ground black pepper
3 tablespoons apple-cider vinegar

Preheat the oven to 180C. Place the onions, garlic, pears, sweet potato, tomatoes, maple syrup, salt, pepper and vinegar into a large casserole dish and mix well. Add the lentils, and stir them through. Cover the dish, or place tin foil over it, and bake for at least half an hour, until the sweet potato has softened. Uncover, and bake for another ten minutes. Adjust the seasonings if necessary. Serve with rice or salad.

Mediterranean Vegetables Baked with Lentils

We eat a lot of lentils in our home. Why? Because they're a fabulous source of nutrition, and despite the jokes laid at their humble tootsies, they are just so versatile. I know that even when I'm overdue to do a grocery shop, if I spy a jar of lentils still on the dresser I know for sure that we're not going to starve.

5 cups cooked Puy lentils
6 peppers, chopped
1 courgette, chopped
1 red onion, chopped
4 tomatoes, chopped
1 teaspoon dried Italian herbs
½ teaspoon smoked paprika
1 teaspoon salt
Generous grinding of coarse black pepper
180g chargrilled red-pepper paste
180g water

Apart from the lentils, red pepper paste and water, place all ingredients into a casserole dish, and drizzle well with olive oil. Bake for 30 minutes at 200C.

Stir halfway through cooking. After half an hour, remove from the oven and mix through the final three ingredients. Bake for another ten minutes.

Serve with salad and brown-rice spaghetti.

Apricot and Black Bean Ragoût

There's just something so exotic, and if I'm honest, a tad naughty about adding fruit to a savoury dish. Perhaps because my Mum drilled it into me to eat fruits separately to all other foods so they can digest quickly in the way Nature intended (which is actually true). So, here's my bad-girl recipe. Sorry, Mum! I still love you.

6 dried apricots, pitted
4 prunes, pitted
Olive oil
1 onion, chopped
3 cloves garlic, chopped
2 teaspoons dried oregano
1 cup red pepper, chopped
1 can tomatoes, chopped
2 cups sweet potatoes, chopped
1 cup frozen corn kernels
2 cups cooked black beans
Salt and pepper to taste

Cover the fruit in boiling water, and soak for a few hours, then drain and chop. Keep the liquid to one side.

Preheat the oven to 180C.

Sauté the onion, garlic, and oregano for a few minutes, then add the pepper and tomatoes. Add the sweet potato, liquid from the fruit, and bring to the boil. Simmer for twenty minutes. Add the corn and beans, then season and simmer. Serve over the grain of your choice.

Courgette and Aubergine Bake

It's a balmy day in the Mediterranean. An old man, face weather-worn from decades of sunshine, strums his mandolin. He leans against the wall, in his white jeans, his silver stubble glistening in the sunshine, while humming a sailor's ballad. There's a peaceful ambience on the sea breeze as you sit down to eat this traditional dish.

In my reality, it's more likely that I'm eating it on a bitterly cold English night while snuggling up closely to the woodstove before I die of frostbite!

1 can tomatoes, chopped
1 tablespoon tomato paste
Olive oil
4 cloves garlic, chopped
Juice of 1 lemon
Pinch of cinnamon
1 potato, sliced
1 onion, sliced
1 red pepper, sliced
1 courgette, sliced
1 aubergine, sliced
Sea salt and pepper to taste
Handful fresh parsley, chopped
Handful fresh oregano, chopped

Preheat the oven to 220C. Mix the tomatoes, tomato paste, a little olive oil, garlic, cinnamon and lemon juice. Place the potato slices into the base of a deep casserole dish. Place about a third of the tomato mixture on top, then place the onion, then more sauce. Layer on the pepper, then sauce, the courgette, then aubergine, finishing with any sauce that's left. Sprinkle a little salt and pepper, drizzle with olive oil, and bake for about 30 minutes or until the aubergine is cooked. Garnish with fresh herbs.

Zen. . . does not confuse
spirituality with thinking about God
while one is peeling potatoes.

Zen spirituality is just to peel the potatoes.

Alan W. Watts, 'The Way of Zen', 1957

Brazilian Bean Stew

Brazilian cuisine is heavily influenced by Amerindian, European and African cultures. Like a magpie, it searches out the most interesting pieces and gathers them unto itself.

1 cup tomato juice
1½ cups brown rice
2 tablespoons olive oil
1 large onion, finely chopped
2 cloves garlic, finely chopped
3 medium sweet potatoes, peeled and cut into small cubes
4 cups cooked black beans, drained and rinsed
1 red pepper, finely chopped
1 cup chopped ripe tomatoes
1 small fresh green chilli
¼ cup chopped fresh coriander
Salt and pepper, to taste

Bring three cups of water and juice to a simmer. Add the rice, and cook gently for about half an hour until the liquid is absorbed.

Meanwhile, sauté the onion and garlic until brown, then add the sweet potatoes and 1½ cups of water. Simmer until the potatoes are tender. Add the chilli, tomatoes, pepper and beans. Simmer for a further fifteen minutes. Stir in the coriander, and adjust the seasonings.

Aubergine Curry

Aubergines are the sponges of the vegetable world, and are fantastic at absorbing flavours. No surprise, then, that it works so beautifully in curry.

2 large aubergines, cut into chunks
1 green pepper, sliced
Olive oil
1 teaspoon mild chilli powder
1 onion, chopped
1 teaspoon black mustard seeds
2 tablespoons curry paste
150g red lentils
450ml vegetable bouillon
Handful of chopped fresh coriander

Heat the oven to 190C. Place the aubergines and pepper into a baking tray, and drizzle with oil and sprinkle with chilli. Bake for about 35 - 45 minutes, until soft, turning if necessary from time to time.

While this is cooking, sauté the onion until soft, then add the mustard seeds, and curry paste. Stir in the uncooked lentils and bouillon. Simmer for twenty minutes then add the aubergine once it has cooked. Stir in fresh coriander. Serve with rice or Indian bread.

Macadamia and Red Pepper Roast

Due to them not being the cheapest nut available here in England, I often just dream about macadamia nuts. I love them as they are, but have fond memories of sultry Australian days refreshed by a good ol' Queensland macadamia-nut ice cream. When I do remember to buy these nuts, this is one of my favourite ways of using them.

Olive oil (for greasing loaf tin)
800g carrots, chopped or grated
1 red onion
3 celery sticks, chopped
4 cloves garlic, chopped
300g macadamia nuts, chopped
3 red peppers, chopped
3 leeks, chopped
3 tablespoons fresh parsley
2 teaspoons lemon juice (fresh)
½ organic lemon, zest
1 inch ginger root, finely grated
3 tablespoons nutritional yeast flakes
½ cup rice flour

Preheat oven to 200C.
Steam the vegetables until tender, then mix with the remaining ingredients (except olive oil). When thoroughly mixed, place into a greased loaf tin, or one lined with baking paper, and bake for one hour. Serve with salad.

Beetroot-Jewelled Butternut Bake

This is such a delightfully coloured regal dish that I simply had to use jewel in the title. Queen Butternut!

Butternut squash (one large or two small)
2 fresh beetroots
100g vegan Greek-style cheese, cut into cubes
2 red onions
Handful black and green olives
Soaked sun-dried tomatoes
Fresh rosemary leaves
Olive oil
3 tablespoons balsamic vinegar
5 tablespoons maple syrup
Salt
Freshly ground black pepper

Preheat the oven to 200C. Cut the butternut in half, and scoop out the seeds and a little of the flesh. Drizzle with a little olive oil and sprinkle with salt and place on a baking tray.

Peel or scrub the beetroots then chop into cubes about 1.5 cm wide. Peel, then cut the red onions in half, and finely slice.

Cut the sundried tomatoes into strips. Place the beetroot cubes, onions, several fresh rosemary leaves, and tomatoes onto a baking tray and drizzle with olive oil, balsamic vinegar, and maple syrup. Sprinkle with salt and pepper.

Bake the beetroot mix and the pumpkin until tender; about 35 - 40 minutes. Remove from the oven and mix the olives, and about 100g of cheese, into the beetroot. Stir, then spoon the mixture into the pumpkin and bake for another five minutes.

You might want to scoop out a bit more pumpkin flesh so the cavity is larger. Add any extra butternut flesh into the beetroot mix. Serve with a leafy green salad.

Sunday Breakfast Lentils

You could have baked beans on toast for breakfast. You could! Or, you could have this...

Olive oil
3 cloves garlic, chopped
2½ cups cooked Puy lentils
2 cups cherry tomatoes
¼ cup organic tomato sauce
¼ cup maple syrup
1 tablespoon balsamic vinegar
1 tablespoon blackstrap molasses
1 red pepper, chopped
¼ red onion, chopped
2 carrots, grated
1 teaspoon smoked paprika
1 teaspoon oregano
Salt
Pepper

Roast the tomatoes and garlic (drizzled with a little olive oil) in a 200C oven for 20 minutes.

Sauté the onion, pepper, and carrots until soft. Add the tomatoes and garlic. Add the remaining ingredients (except the lentils). When cooked, add the lentils and simmer for fifteen minutes.

Serve on toast, polenta, hashbrowns, or a bed of mashed sweet potato.

Spaghetti and Meatballs

Who said you can't have spaghetti and meatballs if you're vegan and gluten free? Just watch me!

3 cups cooked red lentils, drained
1½ cup breadcrumbs or stuffing mix
2 tablespoons peanut butter (or nut/seed butter of choice)
1 teaspoon Italian herbs
1 teaspoon salt
1 teaspoon cumin
1 teaspoon coarse-ground black pepper
½ teaspoon onion powder

Sauce
2 cups pasatta (sieved tomatoes)
2 teaspoons smoked paprika
1 teaspoon Italian herbs
½ teaspoon salt
3 tablespoons maple syrup
1 cup water

Spaghetti

Cook the lentils until soft, drain excess liquid, then process with the other meatball ingredients. Roll into small balls, and bake at 190C for 25 minutes until golden brown.

Meanwhile, heat the sauce ingredients, and cook the spaghetti. When ready to serve, gently stir the balls into the sauce, then ladle over the spaghetti. Garnish with fresh parsley, and cheese, if desired.

White Bean and Sage Roast

500g cooked white beans
100g cooked rice (or quinoa)
3 tablespoons tomato paste
2 teaspoons smoked paprika
1 teaspoon vegetable bouillon powder
2 tablespoons tamari
1 tablespoon dried-onion flakes
1 tablespoon dried sage
100g brown-rice flour
50g chickpea flour
Salt and black pepper to taste

Place the beans and rice in a food processor and blend until smooth, then add the rest of the ingredients. Place into a lined loaf tin. Bake for 45 minutes at 185C.

Sweet Potato and Brazil Nut Roast

If you're looking for something special for your Christmas meal, make this your feature dish. It's delicious at any time of year, though.

1 large sweet potato, grated
1 cup Brazil nuts, chopped
1 red pepper, chopped
200g breadcrumbs
1 red onion, chopped
2 cloves garlic, chopped
1 cup cheese, grated
1 cup fresh parsley, chopped
1 tablespoon bouillon powder
1 tablespoon Italian herbs
¼ cup water, approximately

Place all ingredients (except breadcrumbs and water) into a food processor and mix until the nuts are a lot smaller. Add the breadcrumbs, and about ¼ - ½ cup of water, and mix some more.

Place into paper muffin cups, and bake at 200C for 15-20 minutes, or into a loaf tin and bake for 30 minutes.

Serving suggestion:
Serve with stir-fried slices of Brussels sprouts, yellow pepper, a few chopped tomatoes and a pinch of fennel seeds.

Chestnut and Feta Roast

This makes an absolutely gorgeous feature for a Christmas celebration. It's earthy, savoury, and ever so scrummy. Don't be fooled by the simplicity of this dish.

2 cups Brazil nuts
2 leeks, thinly sliced
2 red peppers, chopped
400g chestnuts, chopped
2 cloves garlic, chopped
1 tablespoon Italian herbs
2 tablespoons bouillon powder
1 tablespoon sesame seeds
100g breadcrumbs
200g feta (vegan Greek-style cheese)
3 tablespoons flaxseeds
100ml maple syrup
Pinch of dried rosemary

Mix all the ingredients well. Place into a loaf tin, and bake for 45-55 minutes at 190C.

Lasagne

Lasagne, is pronounced *la zarn ya*. The singular piece of pasta is spelled: lasagna. One of the world's oldest types of pasta, they consist of wide, flat sheets, and the dish is made by layering sheets with alternate layers of sauces and other ingredients, traditionally cheese, tomato and meat. It is believed to have its origins in Naples, where it became a familiar dish. Lasagne are always oven baked. The dough for the pasta uses semolina in the south, and flour and eggs in the north. In my recipes, I use gluten-free pasta made from quinoa or rice flour.

When our daughter Beth was a toddler, we would take her to our favourite café in Ponsonby, Auckland (New Zealand), where the chef would cook her up a whole plate of sautéed mushrooms. She'd scoff the lot.

She's no longer a tot. For Beth's 21st birthday, she asked if I'd make her a mushroom lasagne. Well, given mushrooms are probably the one thing I can eat on an almost daily basis, I can assure you it was no hardship.

The great thing about lasagne is that you have a basic template: pasta sheets, cheese or tomato sauce, and white sauce. The vegetable mix can be as varied as some of my favourites: mushroom, slow-roasted Mediterranean vegetables, fennel and tomato, pea, mint and asparagus, spinach and nutmeg with butternut squash.

Mushroom Lasagne

1kg button or mixed mushrooms
7 cloves garlic, roughly chopped
Olive oil
750ml coconut cream
Salt (1-2 two teaspoons)
Pepper (generous pinch or two)
Fresh thyme (about 1 tablespoon or so)
Lasagna sheets
Cheese (optional)

Toss mushrooms, sliced or whole if small, onto a tray with garlic and olive oil, salt, pepper and thyme. Roast for 40 minutes at 200C.

Remove, and add to a bowl with coconut cream. Mix well, and allow to sit for half an hour so the flavours can infuse.

Spread the mushroom and cream sauce between layers of lasagna sheets. Reserve some cream for pouring over the final sheet of pasta or cover with grated cheese. Bake covered, for half an hour or so, then remove cover and bake for five minutes. Use a knife to check that pasta has cooked (some brands of gluten-free pasta take longer than others).

Asparagus Lasagne

1kg asparagus, tough woody ends chopped off
250g grated cheese
Bunch of spring onions, sliced
Salt
Pepper
Six cloves garlic, chopped
1 lemon zest (organic)
1kg frozen peas
Handful of mint
2 teaspoons fresh thyme leaves
500ml soy, rice or coconut cream
500g feta (vegan Greek-style)
500ml vegetable bouillon
Lasagna sheets
1 tablespoon plain flour
1-2 cups milk, unsweetened

Fry the asparagus in olive oil, fresh thyme and salt for a few minutes. Add the peas and bouillon and simmer until the liquid has mostly evaporated. Add the cream and mint, and mix well. Place the lasagna sheets in a greased casserole dish. Cover with grated cheese, then the asparagus mix. Crumble the feta on top. Repeat layers until everything is used up. Create a white sauce for the top by sautéing the flour in a little oil in a pan, then adding the milk slowly until a sauce forms. Whisk continuously. Season with salt and pepper, then spread over the top of the lasagne, and cover. Bake for about half an hour at 200C (until the lasagna sheets are tender).

Mediterranean Vegetable Lasagne

As for the mushroom lasagne recipe, but instead of mushrooms, slow-roast:

2 courgettes, sliced
4 red peppers, sliced
1 aubergine, chopped
10 cherry tomatoes
5 cloves garlic
Olive oil
Salt
Black pepper

Lasagna sheets
500ml coconut cream
Cheese

Drizzle vegetables and seasonings well with olive oil and sprinkle with salt and pepper. Bake for 40 minutes. Stir halfway through.

You can make a rich tomato sauce (try Mystic Sauce from The Mystic Cookfire), then layer vegetables and sauce between lasagna sheets. Top with cheese, if desired, and bake at 180C for 30 minutes or until pasta is tender.

Butternut and Sage Lasagne

There's a large healthy sage bush in my garden.

According to folklore, anyone who has sage planted in their garden is reputed to do well in business.

Sage has long been revered, and is thought to have sacred qualities. Traditionally, sage was believed to aid conception, treat the plague, protect against witchcraft and spells, as well as enhance memory. As a herb, it's a valuable source of vitamin A, iron, potassium, and calcium.

6 cups butternut squash, peeled and cubed
2 tablespoons olive oil
¼ cup chopped fresh sage
6 garlic cloves, left whole
1 teaspoon sea salt
Pinch of black pepper

Cheese-style layer
2 cups firm tofu
¼ cup nutritional yeast flakes
1 teaspoon garlic powder
1 teaspoon dried dill
1 teaspoon sea salt
1 tablespoon apple-cider vinegar

White Sauce
¼ cup olive oil
1 onion, finely chopped
4 tablespoons flour
4 cups unsweetened milk

Pinch of salt
Two pinches of fresh black pepper
Small pinch of smoked paprika

Preheat oven to 205C.

Mix the first list of ingredients, and bake on a baking tray for half an hour. Turn halfway through. When cooked, mash with a fork. Put to one side.

Place the 'cheese' ingredients in a food processor and mix for one minute, and set to one side.

From the final list of ingredients, sauté the onion in the oil for a few minutes, then add the flour. Stir for a few minutes, then add the milk. Whisk the whole time, then bring to the boil. Turn down and simmer. When the sauce has thickened, add smoked paprika, salt and pepper.

Heat the oven to 175C.
At the bottom of the baking dish, place half the white sauce, then the lasagna sheets, then some cheese sauce, then lasagna sheets, then pumpkin mix. Repeat layers until the ingredients are used up. Cover with tin foil, and bake for forty minutes. Remove the foil and bake uncovered for another 15 minutes.

If you have spare sage leaves, fry them in a little olive oil or vegan butter until crisp, and serve on top of the lasagne.

Roast Fennel and Tomato Lasagne

This is my absolute favourite way to eat fennel!

6 fennel bulbs, thinly sliced
3 punnets cherry tomatoes
1 head garlic, left whole and unpeeled
Lasagna sheets
Sea salt
Pepper
500ml soya (or other plant-based) cream, unsweetened
Olive oil

Place the fennel on a baking tray, and the tomatoes and garlic on another baking tray, and drizzle both with olive oil, and sprinkle with salt and pepper. Bake the fennel at 200C for about 30 minutes, and the tomatoes and garlic for about 25 minutes.

Peel the garlic (the insides should just pop out!) Place the tomatoes and garlic into a bowl and mash. Add the cream and stir through.

Place the lasagna sheets into a casserole dish, and cover with the fennel. Place another layer of lasagna, then cover with the tomato mixture. If you use a narrow lasagne dish you will get a few layers. Make sure the top layer of lasagne is well covered in the tomato sauce. Bake, covered, for about half an hour at 200C.

Serve with a luscious salad.

Love Notes

Burgers, falafel, fritters and pizza

Mint and Pea Fritters

Mint promotes digestion, improves oral health, is said to prevent cancer, support the memory, and clear congestion of the throat, lungs and nose.

2 tablespoons coconut or other plant yoghurt
600g frozen peas, partly mashed
3 tablespoons chia seeds
1 cup rice flour
¾ cup water
Handful chopped parsley
Handful chopped fresh mint
Zest of a lime
1 tablespoon bouillon powder
1 teaspoon coarse-ground black pepper
1-2 teaspoons sea salt

Beat the yoghurt and chia seeds. Add the remaining ingredients, and mix well. Scoop about 2 tablespoons for each fritter.

Gently fry in olive or coconut oil for a few minutes until cooked on both sides.

Herb and Almond Burgers

Olive oil
3 cloves garlic, chopped
Sea salt
1 onion, chopped
2 carrots, grated
1 cup ground almonds
2 tablespoons almond butter
Generous pinch of dried Italian herbs
Handful fresh parsley, chopped
1 teaspoon fresh thyme leaves
2 cups bread crumbs
Water

Sauté the onions, garlic and a little salt for a few minutes, then add the carrot, and cook for a few more minutes.

Mix the vegetables with the remaining ingredients, and then add the water, mixing well. Shape into burgers, and then gently fry for a few minutes on each side. Serve with salad and chutney.

Fennel and Beetroot Croquettes

If you're looking to get more of the earth element into your diet, look no further. Beetroot is amazing! It's a real blood cleanser, and so rich in nutrients. It is one of those vegetables that's been around for such a long time, originating along the coastlines of North Africa. Originally eaten for its leaves, the root wasn't cultivated until ancient Roman times.

Napoleon declared beets a source of sugar after the Brits restricted access to sugar cane. Amongst beetroot's health benefits are that it lowers blood pressure, boosts stamina, aids detoxification, fights inflammation, and has anti-cancer properties.

1 onion, chopped
2 cloves garlic, chopped
1 cup mushrooms
2 beetroots, grated
½ cup raw Brazil nuts
1 cup cooked black beans
2 tablespoons ground flax seeds
1 tablespoon nutritional yeast flakes
2 teaspoons oregano
1 teaspoon smoked paprika
1 teaspoon salt
½ teaspoon fennel seeds
Pinch of freshly ground black pepper
Pinch of smoked paprika

Chop nuts in a processor, then place in a mixing bowl. Add grated beetroot to the food processor, and add mushrooms, garlic, and onion, and process for a minute. Add the beans, and then the remaining ingredients, and mix until combined. Form into croquettes the size of golf balls, then bake on a greased tray at 175C for 30 minutes.

Carrot and Ginger Fritters

Another fab earth element recipe.

2 tablespoons ground flaxseeds
5 tablespoons water
2 cups carrots, grated
1 cup courgettes, grated
2 spring onions, sliced
2 tablespoons parsley, chopped
2 cloves garlic, finely chopped
3 tablespoons chickpea flour (also known as gram or besan)
1 teaspoon cumin
Pinch of turmeric
2 inches ginger root, finely grated
Pinch of salt
Olive oil

Mix together the flaxseeds and water and leave until thickened. Combine the rest of the ingredients (apart from the oil), and then stir the flax mix in.

Drizzle the oil in a pan, and heat to medium. For each fritter, place a ladle of batter into the pan. Fry for five minutes on each side.

Serve with leafy or steamed greens.

A Carrot a Day Keeps PMT Away!

The majority of Western women experience premenstrual tension, infertility, mood disorders, menopausal problems, and for men there can be erectile dysfunction, moobs (man boobs) and poor muscle tone, all caused by oestrogen dominance. This can be caused by emotional, physical or environmental stress. Did you know that you can help to detox excess oestrogen by eating a raw carrot each day? The fibre in carrots absorbs the oestrogen and sweeps it out of the body.

Irish Potato Cakes

This is dedicated to my trio of lovely friends who live in Ireland: Siobhán, Mandy and Claire. I love you all!

4 large sweet potatoes, chopped
1 red onion, chopped
1 cup red cabbage, chopped
½ cup fresh parsley, chopped
1 teaspoon salt
2 tablespoon nutritional yeast flakes
1/3 cup chickpea flour
Pinch smoked paprika
½ cup water
Olive or coconut oil

Preheat oven to 220C. Sauté the onion, potatoes and cabbage for a few minutes, then add water, and cover the saucepan. Simmer for about 10 minutes, until the potatoes are tender.

Mash the vegetables, and add the remaining ingredients (except oil). Form into cakes the size of your palm. Bake on a baking sheet, sprinkled with the oil, for about ten minutes on each side until crispy brown.

Laughter is brightest,
in the place where the food is.
Irish proverb

Baked Black-Bean Falafel
with Papaya and Mint Salsa

My mum had a pawpaw tree (papaya) in the sun-drenched courtyard of my childhood home. Living in the far north of England now, I rarely (and sadly) get to taste a truly ripe tropical fruit.

700g cooked black beans
3 cups cooked quinoa
8 cloves garlic, chopped
½ red onion, chopped
Pinch of hot chilli powder
10 tablespoons chickpea flour
Salt to taste (1 to 2 teaspoons)
Freshly ground black pepper (½ teaspoon)

Preheat the oven to 170C. Place the garlic, onion, chilli powder and black beans into a food processor and mix well. Add the quinoa, chickpea flour and salt and pepper. Mix well. With damp hands, shape into falafel, about the size of a walnut shell. Bake for half an hour on a greased tray or baking sheet. These can also be shallow fried, if preferred.

Papaya and Mint Salsa
1 papaya (pawpaw), finely chopped
1 large ripe tomato, finely chopped
½ lime, finely grated zest; and ½ lime, juice
¼ red onion, finely chopped
Dash of chilli powder

Combine all the ingredients.

Sesame and Courgette Fritters

Eaten by humans for over five-thousand years, sesame seeds are a fabulous source of calcium, zinc, copper, manganese and magnesium. Courgettes and sesame seeds fall under the 'fruit' or fire element and are great for warming the metabolism.

2 courgettes, chopped
1 onion, chopped
1 clove garlic, chopped
2 tablespoons fresh parsley
Generous pinch of salt
¼ teaspoon baking powder
¼ teaspoon black pepper
½ cup rice flour
¼ cup nutritional yeast flakes
3 tablespoons ground flax seeds
5 tablespoons sesame seeds
Olive or sesame seed oil

Preheat the oven to 220C. Line a baking tray with a baking sheet and a drizzle of olive or sesame oil. Mix the onion, garlic, courgettes and parsley in a food processor, then place in a bowl with the dry ingredients (only half of the sesame seeds).

Mix well, then form into balls the size of golf balls and scatter the rest of the sesame seeds on top. Place on a baking sheet, and bake for ten minutes on each side.

Serve with a sauce of your choice, such as sweet chilli sauce.

Garlicky Butternut Burgers

I simply adore the vibrant colour of butternut squash!
In colour therapy, orange regulates the metabolism and
circulation. It's associated with the spleen chakra.

Orange is used to stimulate the thyroid gland. It's also a
respiratory stimulant, and the vibrational hue expands
the lungs. Through colour healing, it is used to foster
joy and happiness, so is key in treating hypothyroidism
(low thyroid), depression, bronchitis, asthma, and lung
and kidney ailments.

1 tablespoon ground flax seeds
1 large onion, chopped
4 cloves garlic, chopped
1 cup polenta, uncooked
1 teaspoon smoked paprika
½ teaspoon dried herbs
1-2 teaspoons salt (to taste)
1 teaspoon ground black pepper
3 cups mashed butternut squash, cooled
2 cups cooked quinoa
Olive or coconut oil

Mix the flax seeds with a few tablespoons of water.
Heat the oil in a pan and fry the onion until clear, then
add the garlic, and cook for a few minutes. Add the
flax mix, polenta and seasonings.

Remove from the heat and add quinoa and butternut.
Mix well. Form into burgers with your hands, and
put on a plate and refrigerate for at least half an hour.
Don't skip the chilling process.

Cook the burgers in olive or coconut oil on medium heat, and turn over once a crust has been formed. This takes about five minutes. Serve with salad or steamed vegetables.

One cannot think well, love well, sleep well,
if one has not dined well.
Virginia Woolf

Sweet Potato and Red Onion Falafel

Really, sweet potato should be considered a superfood such is its benefit to the immune system: beta carotene is a major antioxidant, and in sweet potatoes is enhanced with C and B-complex vitamins, iron and phosphorus. As with white potatoes, there is no end to the ways you can cook them.

2 baked sweet potatoes, peeled after cooking
1 red onion, chopped
2 cloves garlic, chopped
¼ cup fresh parsley
Salt
1 can chickpeas
1 tablespoon apple-cider vinegar
1 teaspoon cumin
1 teaspoon garam masala
¼ teaspoon cayenne
1 cup breadcrumbs
1 cup polenta
Olive or coconut oil

Process the chickpeas, onion, garlic, parsley, salt, sweet potatoes, spices, until mixed well. Add the apple-cider vinegar. Mix again. Move the contents to a bowl, then add the crumbs. Refrigerate for a few hours, then shape into falafel balls. Roll in the uncooked polenta.

Fry on high heat in a pan for a few minutes, until golden on each side.

White Bean and Dill Burgers

½ *cup oats*
2 cups fresh chopped spinach
2 cups white beans, drained and rinsed
2 spring onions, finely chopped
1 tablespoon fresh dill, finely chopped
2 tablespoons vegetable bouillon powder
Pinch ground cumin
Salt and freshly ground pepper to taste
Olive oil

Combine the oats and one cup of boiling water, and leave to stand for about five minutes. Mash the beans, and add to the oats once they're ready. Add the rest of the ingredients, and mix well.

In a pan with hot oil, place a ladle per burger, and cook on both sides until brown. This is lovely served with mashed sweet potato, green salad or steamed vegetables.

Carrot and Nutmeg Fritters

2 teaspoons ground flaxseeds
½ cup water
2 large courgettes, grated
1 sweet potato, grated
1 carrot, grated
1 onion, chopped
Handful of fresh parsley
1 tablespoon organic lemon zest
½ cup breadcrumbs
½ cup plain flour
1 teaspoon baking powder
1 teaspoon salt
2 pinches freshly ground black pepper
Generous pinch of nutmeg
Olive or coconut oil for frying

Allow the flaxseeds to sit in water for about ten minutes. Drain the grated the vegetables, and chop the onion. Add the remaining ingredients (apart from the flour) to a bowl with the grated vegetables, then add the flaxseeds, and combine. Finally, add the flour. Chill the mixture in the fridge for half an hour.

Form into small balls, and fry for a few minutes on each side until golden brown. Add more oil during cooking if necessary.

Earthy Walnut and Lentil Burgers

Walnuts are a fabulous source of protein and omega-3 fatty acids, and are definitely something worth eating each day. Just a quarter of a cup will provide you with 100% of the daily recommended amount of omega-3 fats, as well as molybdenum, biotin and copper. Walnuts also offer vascular benefits to people with heart disease, and contain unique antioxidants that are available in only a few foods. They're also recommended for male fertility as they can improve sperm quality.

Shaped like the brain, for good reason, they're known homeopathically in the doctrine of signatures as a brain food. It was the 17th-century herbalist, William Coles, who said they were good for treating head ailments. Modern science backs this up. The nutritional element in walnuts is essential for healthy brain function.

1 cup quinoa, cooked
2 cups cooked Puy lentils
1 onion, chopped
1 clove garlic, chopped
1 sweet potato, chopped
Generous handful of walnuts, chopped
½ cup tomato paste
1 tablespoon mustard
3 tablespoons flax seeds, ground
1 teaspoon sea salt
Pinch of smoked paprika
Pinch of cayenne pepper
Pinch coarse-ground black pepper
1 cup polenta

Preheat oven to 230C. Line a tray with baking paper and a drizzle of olive oil.

In a food processor, combine the onion, garlic, sweet potato, and walnuts. Process. Add the quinoa and lentils, and mix. Move to a bowl, then add the tomato paste, and seasonings. Add the polenta, and mix well, then form into patties.

Arrange on a baking tray and drizzle with a little olive oil, and then bake for twenty minutes. Turn over, and bake for another twenty minutes.

Zen proverb:
"When walking, walk.
When eating, eat."

Hash Browns for Eliza

When my daughter Eliza moved from vegetarianism to veganism, one of her great joys was that she could still eat hash browns! Here's a healthier version than you'll find when you're out and about.

2 cups potatoes, skin on, roughly chopped
2 cups onion, chopped
2 cups plain flour
1 cup water
2 teaspoons salt
1 teaspoon coarsely ground black pepper
¼ cup courgette, grated
Handful of fresh parsley, chopped (a clever mum always sneaks in greens somewhere! Shhh!)
1 red pepper, chopped

In a food processor, mix the vegetables until roughly chopped, then add the remaining ingredients and mix again.

To fry: use a ladleful per hash brown, and cook for several minutes (in olive or coconut oil) on each side. Alternatively, if you want to avoid frying, thicken the mix with some polenta, if needed, and then bake for 20 minutes at 200C.

Quinoa Pizza Crust

This is such a beautifully light pizza base.

*2 cups quinoa, soaked for at least 8 hours, rinsed and
drained*
1 cup water
4 tablespoons coconut oil
Two pinches of salt
4 cloves garlic, sliced
2 tablespoons dried Italian herbs
2 tablespoons nutritional yeast

Soak the quinoa in water overnight. Rinse and drain
the quinoa. Place all the ingredients in a food processor
and mix until it becomes a batter. Add more water, if
needed.

Preheat your oven to 230C.

Line a pizza pan with baking paper. Add the quinoa
batter, and then bake for 20 minutes. Turn over, and
bake for ten minutes on the other side until crispy and
brown. Add your toppings.

Suggested toppings: mushrooms, tomatoes, crushed
pineapple, olives, roast peppers, sauce (see Mystic
Sauce, from my recipe book The Mystic Cookfire),
vegan cheese.

Heat for about five minutes in the oven. Just before
serving, rip fresh basil leaves over the top.

Socca Pizza

Socca pizza is one of my favourites. It's a flatbread originating in the south of France. Made from chickpea flour, it's rich in fibre, minerals, vitamins and proteins.

3 cups chickpea flour
Salt and pepper to taste
1½ teaspoons chopped fresh thyme
9 tablespoons olive oil
3 cups water
3 tablespoons coconut oil

Combine the chickpea flour with the salt, pepper, and thyme. Add the olive oil, then the water. Mix well to form a doughy batter.

Leave overnight, if possible (at room temperature) or for a few hours. Keep covered.

Preheat the oven to 205C. Heat a cast-iron skillet in the oven, then remove to add the coconut oil. Pour in one third of the batter, and bake for 8 to 10 minutes. Turn over, and bake for another ten minutes.

Repeat the process for another two pizzas. Keep the cooked ones somewhere warm.

Polenta Pizza

This is such a lovely way to create a pizza base, and if you have any left over is it totally gorgeous eaten cold the next day.

Packet of polenta 250g
1 teaspoon Italian herbs
1 tablespoon olive oil
Pinch of salt
Pinch of ground black pepper
Boiling water

Cook instant polenta, as per packet instructions, including the seasonings. Once cooked, spread out on a pizza tray (I use baking paper underneath). I leave it for an hour or so (optional) to allow it to set some more. Top with a chargrilled red-pepper sauce, and your favourite pizza toppings. Bake for 15 minutes at 200C. Allow to sit for five minutes before slicing.

This tastes even more amazing the next day (if you have any left!)

Love Notes

Saucy stuff!

Smokey BBQ Sauce

Cup organic tomato paste
3/4 cup water
2 teaspoons maple syrup
3 tablespoons blackstrap molasses
1 tablespoon apple-cider vinegar
½ teaspoon ground mustard
½ teaspoon onion powder
½ teaspoon smoked paprika
Pinch of sea salt
Pinch of coarse-ground black pepper

Mix all the ingredients in a blender until smooth, then store in a glass jar. Refrigerate or freeze until needed. This will last about a week in the fridge.

White Bean and Cumin Hummus

2 cups cooked white beans
Juice of half a lemon
3 tablespoons tahini
2 cloves garlic
Pinch of salt
Pinch of cumin
A little water to thin

Place all the ingredients in a food processor, and mix until smooth. Refrigerate.

Roast Pumpkin Seed And Nasturtium Pesto

If your sex life needs amping up a notch or two, why not add a handful of pumpkin seeds to your diet each day? They're chock-full of zinc, a trace element that is essential for optimal sex drive. Did you know that a low zinc level can lead to erectile dysfunction? It can also be a factor in eating disorders, as well as a slow and sluggish labour in birthing women. Zinc is important for the proper functioning of the immune system, can control diabetes, and supports a healthy metabolism. I once pointed out to my lovely dentist that the white spots on his fingernails were due to zinc deficiency. He added pumpkin seeds to his breakfast each day, and what do you know? The next time I saw him he proudly showed me his fingernails: no more spots!

1 cup pumpkin seeds
Ten or so large nasturtium leaves
6 cloves garlic, peeled
1½ cups olive oil
1 cup parmesan cheese (vegan)
Salt to taste

Dry-roast the pumpkin seeds in a pan, stirring so they don't burn, and cook until brown. Place to one side.
Place the nasturtium leaves in boiling water for about ten seconds, and then place into a bowl of cold water, and remove. Place the pumpkin seeds and garlic in a food processor, and process for a few seconds. Add the nasturtium leaves, and blend some more. Slowly add the olive oil. Remove from the processor, and then add the cheese and salt. This pesto will last a week or so if refrigerated.

Decadent Creamy Sauce

¼ cup plain flour
¼ cup olive oil
3 cloves garlic, finely chopped
½ cup milk, unsweetened
1 cup water
½ teaspoon salt
2 tablespoons nutritional yeast flakes
1 teaspoon lime juice
1 teaspoon tamari
Black pepper to taste

Heat a little oil in a pan, then add the flour and stir for about half a minute at low heat. This will thicken. Add the garlic, and cook for a couple more minutes. Add the milk, and keep stirring while it thickens. Now, add the water slowly, whisking the whole time to stop lumps forming and to prevent it getting too thick. Add the rest of the ingredients, and stir gently. It should be smooth, and taste fabulous. This sauce is superb over steamed vegetables or with pasta.

Sweet Ginger and Peanut Sauce

This is absolutely perfect over stir-fried vegetables. Ginger and peanut butter are two of my top-five favourite foods.

½ cup crunchy peanut butter (I use Whole Earth Organic)
2 tablespoons rice mirin (available in speciality section of the supermarket or in health stores)
2 tablespoons tamari
2 tablespoons fresh finely grated ginger root
2 tablespoons maple syrup
¼ cup water

Mix well, and heat gently.

Rosemary Gravy

As a celebrant, I often use rosemary in my ceremonies; that's why I have seven bushes in my garden. This herb represents remembrance. Wedding rings, tied with ribbon to a twig of rosemary, can be passed around to guests at the start of the ceremony to 'warm' the rings and imbue them with a blessing.

At small funerals, I often have a piece of rosemary for each mourner to place on the coffin as they say their final farewell. The scent of rosemary stays with people and fills their hearts with memories of the person they associate it with.

¼ cup flour
¼ cup nutritional yeast flakes
¼ cup olive oil
2¼ cups water
½ teaspoon salt
1 teaspoon crushed rosemary
½ teaspoon turmeric powder
Pinch of coarse-ground black pepper

On a low heat, cook the flour and nutritional yeast for about two minutes (keep stirring). Add the oil, and then whisk to avoid lumps. Add water, then seasonings. Continue to cook on low heat for a few minutes. Velvety and creamy, this is a great sauce to pour over steamed vegetables.

Love Notes

Some people think being vegetarian or vegan is boring. I never feel deprived. Ever. Though, in fairness, if I was raised experiencing vegetables as boiled cabbage, or boiled everything, maybe I would also feel like that. If I sneak back into the dark, deep recesses of my memory banks to when I used to stay at friends' houses as a kid, three boiled veg at the side of a plate is exactly what they had.

My mother's cooking, however, was absolutely delicious, vibrant and colourful!

Voluptuous vegetables

Roast Cauliflower and Red Onion with Ginger and Peanut Butter Sauce

2 heads cauliflower (1 large, or 2 small), cut into florets
2 cans chickpeas, rinsed well and drained
1 red onion, peeled and cut into wedges
2 cloves garlic, chopped
Olive or coconut oil
1 tablespoon turmeric

Combine the ingredients in a casserole dish, and cook at 200C for about 30 minutes, stirring halfway through, or until the cauliflower is tender and roasted.

Ginger and Peanut Butter Sauce
½ cup crunchy peanut butter
2 tablespoons tamari
2 tablespoons fresh finely grated ginger root
2 tablespoons maple syrup
2 tablespoons rice mirin
¼ cup water

Mix well, and heat gently. Pour over the cauliflower mix when serving.

Serving Suggestion
150g brown rice
Boiling water
2 tablespoons tamari
2 handfuls baby spinach leaves
Sea salt
Coarse-ground black pepper

Cook the rice until fluffy and the water has been absorbed.

To the cooked rice, add the tamari and spinach and mix through. When the leaves have wilted, put the rice into the serving bowls. Top with the cauliflower, and drizzle the sauce over.

Marinated Picnic Vegetables

Store these in a glass Kilner jar and take along on a picnic. No need for cutlery! Use your fingers. Go on, I dare you.

Marinade
½ cup good-quality olive oil
½ cup sunflower oil
¼ cup red-wine vinegar
1 tablespoon dried Italian herbs
2 tablespoons maple syrup
1 clove garlic, finely chopped
1 inch of ginger root, finely grated

Vegetables
2 cups broccoli florets
2 cups cauliflower florets
1 cup carrot sticks
1 cup small button mushrooms, cut in half

Whisk the marinade ingredients and pour into a glass jar. Add the vegetables, and turn upside down a few times till they're well coated. Leave overnight, turning a few times before serving.

Mushroom-Stuffed Peppers

1 onion
1 cup mushrooms, finely chopped
1 jalapeño pepper, finely chopped
2 cups black beans, cooked
2 cups corn kernels
2 cups tomatoes, finely chopped
1 teaspoon smoked paprika
Pinch of chilli powder
1 teaspoon salt
5 red bell peppers

Sauté the onion until it softens, then add the mushrooms and jalapeño. Once the mushrooms have softened, add the remaining ingredients (except the peppers) and simmer for ten minutes.

Preheat the oven to 205C. Remove the stems and seeds from the peppers, and then stand them upright in an oiled baking dish (slice a little off the bottom if they're not standing). Fill each pepper with the mushroom mix.

Bake for about 40 minutes. Garnish with fresh coriander or parsley.

Butternut and Thyme Risotto

I never fail to be charmed by the exotic citrusy scent of fresh thyme. My fingers brush the leaves as I walk by my herb garden, and I am at once sated by this simple pleasure in my life.

1 butternut squash, peeled and cut into cubes
5-6 cups vegetable bouillon
1 tablespoon olive oil
1 red onion, chopped
2 cups Arborio rice, rinsed
¼ cup rice mirin
¼ cup water
2 tablespoons fresh thyme
Tamari

Simmer the vegetable bouillon.

In a pan, sauté the onion in olive oil. After a few minutes, add a sprinkle of tamari. Add the rice, and keep stirring. Add the mirin and water, and keep cooking and stirring until the liquid has absorbed.

Add the bouillon to rice, stirring frequently, and cook until the rice is creamy and tender. Add the thyme leaves. Cook gently for another 20 minutes.

Mediterranean Vegetables
with Mashed Butter Beans

There's something extremely satisfying about both the simplicity and scrumptiousness of this dish.

2 red peppers, deseeded and sliced into thick chunks
2 aubergines, sliced lengthways
4 courgettes, sliced lengthways
3 ripe tomatoes, left whole
4 tablespoons olive oil
Salt

For the beans
2 cups cooked butter beans
1 clove garlic, finely chopped
100ml vegetable bouillon
Coarse-ground black pepper
1 tablespoon chopped coriander

Roast the vegetables in the oven for about 25-30 minutes at 200C.

For the mash, place the beans, garlic and stock into a pan and simmer for ten minutes. Mash. Add a little water if it seems too thick.

Place the bean mash on each plate, then place vegetables on top. Garnish with coriander, and sprinkle a pinch of two of black pepper on top.

Mushroom Pakoras

Mushrooms are just one of those foods that people either love or hate. Me, I love 'em! I grew up on a horse stud in rural Queensland, Australia. Whenever it rained, which actually wasn't that often, mushrooms would sprout up everywhere. My siblings and I would go out with buckets and collect them. My mother's mushroom and parsley soup was nothing short of perfection. Although it is one of my favourite childhood food memories, the truth is that whenever I eat mushrooms, no matter how they're cooked, I am always right back there on the farm, barefoot and chasing wild mushrooms.

The addition of chickpea flour makes this a great way to get some protein. Serve these alongside a salad or to accompany a soup or rice, or for a dinner party as a starter, or simply on their own for no other reason than that they are yum!

2 cups chickpea flour (also known as gram or besan flour)
1 teaspoon salt
Pinch of cumin
Pinch of dried coriander
Pinch of turmeric
Pinch of cayenne
1 teaspoon finely grated ginger
1 onion, chopped
10 mushrooms, chopped
Handful fresh coriander leaves
Olive or coconut oil for cooking

Mix the flour and spices well in a bowl. Slowly add warm water and whisk to form a thick batter. Add the rest of the ingredients, and leave to sit for about half an hour to allow the spices to release their flavours.

These can be baked or fried.

To bake, preheat the oven to 220C. Use a baking sheet or lightly grease a tray. Bake for 12 minutes or so.

To fry, cook in oil on medium heat. Allow about a tablespoon per pakora. Fry for about five minutes on each side. When cooked, place on paper towels so the oil can absorb.

Asparagus with Mushroom Quinoa

Spring is such an amazing time in the garden. There's that sense of possibility and faith that everything will come to fruition. One of the first foods of the season is asparagus. In my early twenties, whilst travelling, I worked on an asparagus farm in Hawke's Bay New Zealand. Asparagus is amazing! You cut a spear, and lo and behold, the next day it's as if you'd never been there. Yes, they grow that quickly!

Olive oil
300g fresh asparagus
1 large fresh beetroot, thinly sliced
1 leek, sliced
1 cup quinoa
1 to 2 cups water
2 mushrooms, sliced
1 teaspoon sea salt
1 tablespoon balsamic vinegar
Pinch of smoked paprika
½ teaspoon turmeric
Black pepper

Sauté the leek in oil, then add the mushrooms. Cook for a few minutes, then add the quinoa and water. Bring to the boil. Cover, and simmer for 20 minutes. The quinoa should be fluffy. The water should have been absorbed by this time. Sauté the beetroot, with a little salt. When brown, place on a plate. Sauté the asparagus (remove tough ends). Again, add a little sea salt and olive oil. When the quinoa is ready, add the vinegar and spices. Place the vegetables on top.

Cheesy Cauliflower and Sesame Bites

1 large cauliflower, cut into florets
3 tablespoons rice flour
3 tablespoons polenta
1 tablespoon nutritional yeast flakes
1 teaspoon salt
1 tablespoon Italian herbs
2 tablespoons sesame seeds
Pinch of cayenne pepper
Olive oil

Lemon Dressing
1 clove garlic, finely chopped
Salt
½ cup tahini
2 tablespoons lemon juice
Water, as needed
Handful of fresh parsley, finely chopped
Black pepper

Mix the cauliflower with the rest of the ingredients (except for those listed in the dressing). In a heavy-bottomed pan, heat the olive oil and fry the cauliflower, in batches, for about five minutes on each side. When cooked, place on paper towels to absorb the oil.

Dressing
Mix the garlic, salt, tahini and juice, then add water. Keep mixing. Add the pepper and parsley, mix well, and serve alongside the cauliflower bites.

Broccoli with Coconut and Peanut Cream

3 large heads broccoli, chopped into florets
3 cloves garlic, chopped
1 tablespoon olive oil

Coconut and Peanut Cream
1 cup coconut cream
3 tablespoons peanut butter
Pinch of salt
Pinch of coconut sugar or 1 tablespoon maple syrup
1 teaspoon rice vinegar
Pinch of turmeric
Pinch of cayenne pepper

Sauté the broccoli and garlic in olive oil for a few minutes, turning regularly.

Whisk the sauce ingredients over low heat until well combined and heated through, then pour over the broccoli. You might like to serve with quinoa or your favourite grain.

Courgette, Apple and Ginger Chutney

Funny how those little courgettes grow into marrows in a nanosecond. One minute they're babies, then you turn to look at the other vegetables and before you know it there's a glut of big fat marrows staring back at you. What to do? If you've got marrows coming out of your ears, you might like to make this:

4kg marrow or courgettes
2kg apples (I used red gala)
1kg onions
150g salt
4 inches finely grated root ginger
Various spices/herbs: nutmeg, cinnamon, chilli, all spice,
ground ginger, bay leaves (1 teaspoon each)
1kg unrefined brown sugar or coconut sugar
4 litres apple-cider vinegar

Chop the marrow or courgettes into cubes, sprinkle with salt and leave overnight. In the morning, rinse. Put them into a large saucepan with finely chopped onion and apples, plus the spices and a bit of water. Cook until tender, then add the sugar and vinegar. Allow to turn to pulp. You may need to remove some liquid. Sterilise your jars, then fill and seal.

If you can resist, leave for a week or so before eating. Nice served alongside an Indian meal, or with a salad or cheese and bread/crackers.

Thai Tofu with Noodles

For a number of years my father lived in Thailand, and loved to tell me stories of the fresh fruit and vegetables that were so readily available in the streets.

250g King Soba brown-rice noodles
2 aubergines
Olive oil
6 tablespoons Thai green-curry paste
800ml coconut milk
2 tablespoons vegetable bouillon powder
2 packs tofu, sliced in half, then cut into cubes
150g sugar-snap peas, cut in half, lengthwise
1 carrot, cut into thin sticks
2 spring onions, finely chopped
3 to 5 tablespoons maple syrup
Finely grated zest, and juice, of one lime

Garnish
Basil leaves
Freshly ground black pepper (optional)

Cut the aubergines in half, lengthwise, and then into slices about half a centimetre thick. Place on a baking tray and drizzle liberally with olive oil and sprinkle with salt. Bake at 200C for 20 to 30 minutes.

Mix the curry paste with the coconut milk, bouillon powder, peas, spring onions and carrot sticks, and heat. After a few minutes, add the tofu and lime zest and juice. Meanwhile, in another pan, boil your noodles. When cooked, drain, and place into wide or deep bowls. Spoon over your vegetables and sauce, and then garnish.

Mushroom Tapenade

Have I ever mentioned how much I love mushrooms?
One of my top five foods!

2 tablespoons olive oil
3 cloves garlic, finely chopped
1 tablespoon chopped fresh thyme
¼ teaspoon salt
¼ teaspoon pepper
5 cups mushrooms of choice
¼ cup dry white wine (optional) or vegetable bouillon
1/3 cup pitted black olives
1 tablespoon drained capers, rinsed
1 tablespoon chopped fresh parsley

On medium heat, sauté the garlic, thyme, salt and
pepper for a few minutes. Stir the whole time. Add the
mushrooms, and cook for a few more minutes. Keep
stirring. Add the wine, if using (otherwise, bouillon), and
cook until it has evaporated. Add to a food processor,
and mix well. Stores well for a few days in the fridge.
Perfect with crackers.

Sesame-Drenched Asparagus

1 bunch fresh asparagus, tough ends chopped off
1 lemon
¼ cup tahini
½ teaspoon salt
¼ cup sesame seeds
½ teaspoon sesame oil
Freshly ground black pepper, to taste

Preheat the oven to 230C. Place the asparagus on a baking sheet, and drizzle with the sesame oil. Cook for about 20 minutes.

Meanwhile, dry roast the sesame seeds (do not take your eyes off the little beasties or they'll incinerate before you can say 'sesame'. Keep the heat low, and stir the whole time (for a good few minutes). Remove from heat.

Place the cooked asparagus on a plate, and sprinkle lemon juice and drizzle tahini over it. Sprinkle with the salt, pepper and sesame seeds, then toss.

Courgette Polenta Fries

These are so fab!

250g polenta
3 cups water or more, as needed
½ teaspoon salt
½ teaspoon black pepper, or to taste
3 tablespoons nutritional yeast flakes
2 tablespoons Italian herbs
2 cups grated courgette
Olive oil

Cook the polenta as per instructions (I use instant polenta), then when bubbling and thick, add the remaining ingredients (except oil) and stir well. Pour the mix onto a lined baking tray, and allow to cool for 30 minutes, or even refrigerate overnight. This will thicken and set. When ready to cook, cut into fat chips.

Preheat the oven to 230C. Place the chips on lightly oiled baking paper, and bake for 20 minutes. Turn over, and bake for another 15. They should be crispy on the outside, and soft in the middle.

They can be eaten as is, though I like to serve mine with a thick black-bean stew.

My Heavenly Mushrooms

Simple. Quick. Divine. I swoon like a love-struck teenager when I harvest sprigs of fresh thyme from my herb garden, its heady scent accompanying me back to the kitchen, knowing it will partner beautifully with mushrooms.

1kg mushrooms of choice, sliced thinly
4 cloves garlic, finely chopped
2 tablespoons fresh thyme, chopped
1 teaspoon salt or more, to taste
½ teaspoon black pepper
Olive oil

Sauté the mushrooms in a little olive oil for at least five minutes, stirring from time to time. Add the remaining ingredients, and stir while cooking for another five minutes. Now, I could just eat this straight from the pan. However, if I'm in a ladylike mood I'd serve it on a plate with, well, *anything*. Mushrooms don't need to obey food etiquette. They just beg to be eaten.

Corn and Cashew Dumplings
with Mystic Masala Sauce

Dumplings
2 cups potato, unpeeled and chopped
1 cup corn kernels (fresh or frozen)
4 tablespoons toasted cashews, finely chopped
Handful coriander leaves, chopped
½ teaspoon salt
¼ teaspoon turmeric
¼ teaspoon black pepper
Pinch of smoked paprika
½ cup chickpea flour

Mystic Masala sauce
¼ teaspoon garam masala
¼ teaspoon turmeric
1 teaspoon cumin seeds
1 teaspoon fresh ginger, peeled and finely grated
1 onion, chopped finely
Pinch of smoked paprika
1 cup tomatoes, chopped
2 tablespoons cashews, toasted and ground
250ml coconut cream
1 cup water
Salt
Pepper

Toast cashews for five minutes at 220C.

Preheat the oven to 230C. Steam the potatoes and corn, until tender. Mash, and place to one side.

In a pan, sauté the spices for a few minutes and keep

stirring. Add the remaining sauce ingredients. Simmer.

Form a thick dough by combining the potatoes, corn and remaining dumpling ingredients. Form into balls the size of golf balls.

On a baking sheet, place the dumplings a good few centimetres apart. Bake at 230C for about 15 minutes, then turn over and bake for another ten.

To serve, place them on your favourite grain and pour the masala sauce over the top.

Beetroot and Walnut Risotto

This is one of those perfect mid-Winter meals. So earthy.
So deeply nourishing. Enjoy.

4 large beetroots, cut into bite-sized chunks
Olive oil
1 large cauliflower
1 onion, finely chopped
2 cloves garlic, finely chopped
1 cup vegetable bouillon
1 cup walnuts, chopped
Salt and pepper

Preheat the oven to 200C. Place the beetroot in a bowl
and drizzle with the oil, and sprinkle with salt and
pepper. Bake for about 40 minutes.

Place the cauliflower in a food processor and whizz
until it's in small pieces. When done, place in a sieve
until the moisture is removed.

In a pan over medium heat, sauté the onion in a little oil
for several minutes (stirring), then add the garlic. Cook
for a few more minutes, then add the cauliflower and
bouillon. Cook until the liquid has just about absorbed,
then add the beetroot. Cook for a few minutes. Take off
the heat, adjust for seasonings with salt and pepper,
then stir in the chopped walnuts. Serve with a salad.

Roast Cauliflower Tacos

If you're used to having tacos with meat or even beans, think again. This is a lovely light and tasty way of serving them.

1 large cauliflower, broken into florets
1 clove garlic, finely chopped
3 tablespoons olive oil
Salt to taste
Black pepper, to taste
Pinch of cumin

Mix the ingredients together well, then bake for 20-25 minutes until the cauliflower is golden and tender. You want to know what else to do, right? Nothing! Simply place inside the heated taco shells, and add the salad ingredients and cheese (optional) of your choice. Yum, yum, yum!

Broccoli Pakora

1 cup chickpea flour
Two pinches of salt
Pinch of cayenne pepper
1 teaspoon turmeric
1 teaspoon cumin
1 cup finely chopped broccoli
1 cup water

Preheat oven to 230C, and lightly grease a baking sheet.

Mix all the ingredients, except the broccoli, together, ensuring you whisk away any lumps. Add the broccoli to the spicy batter.

Place a large spoonful for each pakora onto a tray. Bake for several minutes on each side until golden. These can be served with rice, quinoa and salad. Or why not try it with a rich tomato chutney for a snack?

Tandoori Roasted Cauliflower

Sometimes I find it hard to believe that I didn't swoon over cauliflower as a child, apart from when it was roasted with potatoes and garlic. This recipe takes good ol' cauli to a whole new level. If you have the time, leave it in the marinade cream overnight. The longer it sits, the longer the spices have to mingle and play.

1 large cauliflower head
2 cups coconut yoghurt (or any plant-based one)
1 tablespoon tandoori or pilau-spice mix
2 pinches of turmeric
1 clove garlic, finely chopped
Pinch of ground ginger
Olive oil (for baking)

Mix all the ingredients, apart from the cauliflower, together until well combined.

Remove the cauliflower leaves and stem, but keep the head of the cauli intact.

Place in a bowl, and cover with the marinade. Refrigerate overnight. When ready to cook, place the cauliflower in a casserole dish which has been lightly greased.

Preheat the oven to 180C. Sprinkle the cauliflower with salt, and bake for 60 or so minutes. If you have any spare marinade, add it to the cauliflower about half way through cooking.

Garlic-Maple Chantenay Carrots

Chantenays are just soooo cute!

1 large onion, finely sliced
1kg Chantenay carrots
4 cloves garlic
Olive oil
2 tablespoons balsamic vinegar
3 tablespoons maple syrup
Salt and freshly ground black pepper

Preheat the oven to 180C. Drizzle the olive oil into a baking dish and then place the onion, carrots and garlic in it. Drizzle with some more olive oil, maple syrup and balsamic, and sprinkle with salt and pepper.

Roast, uncovered, for about 50 minutes, until golden and tender. This can be served hot or cold.

Cauliflower and Date Pilaf

1¼ cups quinoa, rinsed
Olive oil
2 onions, finely chopped
1 cauliflower, broken into small florets
½ cup Medjool dates
Pinch of cumin powder
Pinch of cinnamon
Handful finely chopped coriander
Salt and freshly ground pepper, to taste

Combine the quinoa with a couple of cups of water in a saucepan. Bring to a boil, then cover and simmer gently for 15 minutes, or until the water is absorbed.

Sauté the onions until soft. Add the cauliflower, and a little water. Cover, and cook until tender for a few minutes. When the quinoa is cooked, add the cauliflower, dates, spices and coriander. Mix well, then drizzle some olive oil, and add a pinch of salt and pepper. Serve with salad or baked sweet potatoes.

Love Notes

Sweets

Stewed Berry and Pear Crumble

4 pears
1 cup blueberries
1 cup raspberries
3 tablespoons maple syrup

Crumble
1½ cups oats
1 cup almonds
1 cup pumpkin seeds
4 tablespoons coconut oil
2 tablespoons maple syrup
Pinch of salt

Simmer the berries, 2 cups of water and maple syrup for about twenty minutes.

Cut the pears in half, core, then slice. Add to the berries and simmer.

To make the crumble, place the almonds in the food processor and chop. When done, add to the rest of the crumble ingredients. Bake for half an hour at 160C. Stir every few minutes to avoid burning.

When the crumble is done, place the fruit into serving bowls, and sprinkle the crumble on top.

Cranberry and Almond Slice

3 apples
2 cups dried cranberries
1 cup almonds, soaked in boiling water for a few minutes,
then rinsed
1/3 cup water
2 teaspoons cinnamon
1 teaspoon nutmeg
5 tablespoons maple syrup
2½ cups cooked brown rice
2 flax eggs
½ cup sunflower seeds
2/3 cup plain flour

Preheat the oven to 200C. Chop the apple and put into a food processor. Process for a minute or two then add the spices, flax eggs, water and rice. Process well. Add the flour, cranberries, nuts and seeds and combine.

Place on a lined baking tray. Bake for 20 minutes. Allow to cool before slicing.

Carrot and Cinnamon Balls

2 carrots, chopped
1½ cups walnuts
10 large Medjool dates, pitted
1 cup desiccated coconut
Pinch of nutmeg
Pinch of cinnamon
Pinch of ginger
2 tablespoons oats
2 teaspoons orange zest

Mix the ingredients in a food processor until thoroughly processed. Form into golf-ball sized balls. Serve as they are, or roll in the desiccated coconut. Refrigerate for half an hour.

Banana, Coconut and Chia Bread

1½ cups self-raising flour
Pinch of salt
4 ripe bananas (brown spots on skin), mashed
½ cup desiccated coconut
2 tablespoons chia seeds + 4 tablespoons water
½ cup coconut sugar or maple syrup
¼ cup coconut oil, melted
2 teaspoons vanilla extract

Preheat the oven to 170C. Line a loaf tin with baking paper. Mix the dry ingredients together, and add to the mashed wet ingredients. Combine well and pour into the tin.

Bake for 55 minutes. Allow to cool if you can wait that long. It certainly doesn't happen in our home. Enjoy every single mouthful!

Lemon and Coconut
Rough and Tumble Cookies

I deliberately don't make these into perfect circles, but instead keep the batter a bit wet so they fall all over the tray while cooking. I'm sloppy and slothful at times, but it doesn't detract from the taste one little bit.

¾ cup coconut oil, melted
1 cup coconut sugar
2 teaspoons vanilla essence
2 cups Dove's Farm self-raising flour
2 organic lemons (zest and juice)
1 cup desiccated coconut

Whisk the oil and sugar, then add the remaining ingredients. You may need about ¼ cup water. Mix well. The batter will be wet and sticky. Use about a heaped tablespoon per cookie.

Bake at 180C for 20 minutes. Allow to cool on a wire cooling rack if you possibly can. The scent is intoxicating.

Lime and Mango Cheesecake

Mango: my all-time, life–long, number-one favourite food.

If you can't stand the heat on a Summer's day, be sure to have this gorgeous treat by your side!

Crust
1 cup raw almonds
½ cup Medjool dates
¼ cup desiccated coconut
2 teaspoons vanilla essence
Pinch of salt

Filling
2 ripe mangoes
Half a lime (juice and zest)
½ cup cashew nuts, chopped, and soaked overnight
3 tablespoons coconut oil
5 tablespoons maple syrup
1 cup coconut cream
1 tablespoon fresh mint leaves
½ teaspoon vanilla essence

Whizz all the crust ingredients in a food processor until it forms into crumbs, then divide between four mini-tart pans. Use damp fingers, and press down until it resembles a crust. Leave to one side while you make the filling. Process the mango, cashews (drained), lime juice and zest, coconut oil and cream, mint, vanilla and maple syrup until creamy.

Pour into the crust, and freeze for at least two hours.

Remove from the freezer and leave for only a few minutes before serving. Garnish with fresh mint leaves or lime slices.

Elderberry and Apple Crumble

Comfort food! I enjoy crumbles which don't use flour or butter, but instead I create a topping from seeds, nuts, jumbo porridge oats, and coconut sugar or maple syrup. Once you've mastered the art, there's no end to the variety of crumbles you can create (including savoury options).

3 cups apples
1 cup elderberries (frozen, if out of season)
1 teaspoon cinnamon
Pinch of mixed spice
Pinch of nutmeg
Pinch of ginger
3 tablespoons coconut sugar
Pinch of salt

Crumble:
2 cups rolled oats
¼ cup sunflower seeds
¼ cup pumpkin seeds
6 tablespoons coconut sugar
½ cup coconut oil
2 oranges, freshly squeezed

Slice the apples (if organic, leave the peel on), and place in a baking tray with a little water, spices and coconut sugar. Mix well. Bake at 180C for about 15 minutes, then remove the apples from the oven and add the berries. Make the crumble by mixing the oats, coconut sugar, seeds and melted coconut oil. Place the crumble on top of the fruit, and bake until the topping is golden. This will take about 10-15 minutes.

Rhubarb and Citrus Crumble

Filling
2 cups rhubarb, chopped
¼ cup coconut sugar
1 orange, juice
½ teaspoon ground ginger
¼ teaspoon cinnamon
¼ teaspoon nutmeg
1 tablespoon grated orange zest
1 tablespoon coconut oil

Crumble
½ cup oats
½ cup brown-rice flour
¼ cup sunflower seeds
¼ cup pumpkin seeds
¼ cup toasted coconut flakes
½ cup coconut sugar
½ teaspoon salt
¼ cup coconut oil, melted

Preheat the oven to 190C. Mix the filling ingredients well, then divide into four small oven-proof dishes.

Combine the crumble ingredients well, then sprinkle over the filling mixture. Bake for 40 minutes. The top will be brown, and the fruit juices will bubble up at the sides.

Blueberry and Macadamia Crumble

This is another way to use the utterly glorious, perfect, life-enhancing macadamia.

Filling
2 cups fresh blueberries
¼ cup coconut sugar
2 teaspoons lemon zest (organic)
2 teaspoons water

Crumble
½ cup brown-rice flour
1 cup oats
½ cup coconut or brown sugar
Pinch of salt
½ cup coconut oil, melted
½ cup macadamia nuts, roughly chopped

Preheat the oven to 190C. Mix the filling ingredients. Place in a casserole dish.

Combine the crumble ingredients and spread over the fruit. Bake for half an hour.

No-Cook Raspberry and Pear Crumble

This is adapted from a recipe by my friend, Christina.

1 cup raspberries
4 ripe pears, peeled, cored and chopped

4-5 Medjool dates, pitted
1 tablespoon coconut oil
2 cups ground nuts, cashews, almonds and macadamias
1-2 pinches of cinnamon
Pinch of salt
2-4 tablespoons maple syrup

Arrange the raspberries and chopped pears in a serving dish. Drizzle with the maple syrup (optional).
Sprinkle a dash of cinnamon on top.

In a food processor, blend the nuts, dates, 2 tablespoons of maple syrup and the salt until the mixture resembles breadcrumbs.

Add the coconut oil, cinnamon and salt and blend briefly until you have a good crumble mixture. Arrange the crumble mixture over the fruit and serve.

Raspberry and Vanilla-Infused Apple Crumble

750g raspberries
4 royal gala apples (or apple of choice)
5 tablespoons maple syrup
2 teaspoons vanilla essence
Cinnamon/nutmeg to sprinkle over

Crumble
½ cup sunflower seeds
½ cup desiccated coconut
½ cup coconut sugar
½ cup pumpkin seeds
3 cups oats
¼ cup coconut oil

Slice the apples, and bake in the maple syrup for 20 minutes at 175C.

Melt the coconut oil, and then gently fry the crumble ingredients (not the coconut sugar) for a few minutes. Then, add the sugar.

When the apples have cooked, place the remaining filling ingredients in with them, then top with the crumble and bake for ten minutes.

Raspberry and White-Chocolate Cupcakes

450g self-raising flour
2 teaspoons baking powder
2 flax eggs
100ml coconut oil, melted
200g coconut sugar
3 teaspoons vanilla/almond essence
250ml soya or coconut cream
½ teaspoon apple-cider vinegar
Pinch of salt
400g raspberries
150g white chocolate (vegan), chopped

Preheat the oven to 180C.

Mix the liquid ingredients, then add the dry ones. When mixed, pour into paper cupcake cases. Bake for 20 minutes.

Pear, Vanilla and Nutmeg Cake

800g pear halves
3 tablespoons of maple syrup
500g self-raising flour
1 teaspoon bicarbonate of soda
200g coconut sugar
200ml sunflower oil
500ml apple juice
2 teaspoons pure vanilla essence
Pinch of nutmeg
Coconut or raw brown sugar for sprinkling

Preheat the oven to 180C. Grease a cake tin. Arrange the pears, flat side down, into a flower or star pattern and drizzle with maple syrup.

In a bowl, mix the dry ingredients (except the sugar for sprinkling). Add the liquid ingredients, mix well, and pour over the pears. Bake for 45 minutes.

Remove from the tin, and turn upside down onto an ovenproof plate. Sprinkle the pears with brown sugar, and then place back into the oven and bake for another ten minutes.

Courgette and Chocolate Loaf

400g courgettes, grated
150g coconut oil, melted
3 flax eggs
385g coconut sugar
350g self-raising flour
30g cocoa
1 teaspoon cinnamon
140g walnuts, chopped
2 teaspoon vanilla

Preheat the oven to 175C.

Mix the flax eggs, coconut oil and sugar, then add the remaining ingredients. Put the cake batter into a lined loaf tin, and bake for 50 minutes. If it is humanly possible, allow about 15 minutes to cool.

Apple and Cinnamon Cake

800g royal gala apples, thinly sliced
500g self-raising flour
1 teaspoon bicarbonate of soda
200g coconut sugar
200ml sunflower oil or coconut oil (softened)
500ml soya or other plant milk
Drizzle of maple syrup
1 teaspoon apple-cider vinegar
2 teaspoons pure vanilla essence
½ teaspoon cinnamon
Coconut sugar for sprinkling

Preheat the oven to 180C. Grease two sandwich cake tins or line with baking paper. Arrange the apples slices around the bottom of the tin. Drizzle a little maple syrup over the apples.

Mix the dry ingredients in a bowl (except the sugar for sprinkling). Add the liquids. Mix well and then spread the batter over the apples. Bake for 45 minutes.

Remove from tins, and turn upside down onto an ovenproof baking tray. Sprinkle the apples with coconut sugar. Bake for another ten minutes.

Passionfruit and Mango Cheesecake

As a child, I would spend hours (and I do mean hours) sitting at the bottom of our garden chomping my way through passionfruits that had been hanging lazily off the vine. To this day, I don't bother slicing them in half with a knife because I have the whole 'rip it open with your teeth' thing down to a fine art. However, if I was making this for you I'd use a knife.

Base
2 cups pecans
5 Medjool dates, pitted
2 tablespoons coconut oil

Filling
2 cups cashews (soaked overnight, drained)
1 cup coconut cream
¼ teaspoon vanilla paste
2 tablespoons maple syrup
Pulp of 8 passionfruit
1 ripe fresh mango, blended until smooth

Topping
5 passionfruit pulps

Process the base ingredients, then press into a cake tin and freeze. Mix the filling ingredients until smooth (except the passionfruit). When it is creamy and silky, stir through the passionfruit. Pour the mixture onto the base and freeze. Allow ten minutes to defrost before serving. When ready to serve, spread the remaining passionfruit on top.

Lemon and Coconut Cheesecake

Whether in cupcakes or cheesecakes, lemon and coconut are soulmates!

Base
2 cups almonds
10 Medjool dates, pitted

Filling
2 cups cashews (soaked overnight, drained)
1 cup coconut cream
1 cup lemon juice
Zest of 2 lemons
4 tablespoons maple syrup
1 teaspoon vanilla powder
Extra lemon zest for the top

Process the ingredients to form the base, and then press into a cake tin. Freeze.

Next, mix the filling ingredients until creamy and smooth, pour onto the frozen base, and freeze overnight. Allow it to defrost for about ten minutes before serving.

Sprinkle the zest on top.

Almond and Chocolate Chip Cookies

2½ cups ground almonds
½ teaspoon salt
½ teaspoon bicarbonate of soda
½ cup coconut oil
½ cup maple syrup
1 tablespoon French almond essence
½ cup dark chocolate chips
½ cup sliced almonds

Preheat the oven to 175C, and line a baking tray with parchment paper.

Apart from the chocolate chips and sliced almonds, combine all the ingredients and mix well. Then gently stir the choc chips and almonds through. Allow a tablespoon per cookie, and press down to flatten on the baking sheet.

Bake for fifteen or so minutes.

Banana Cookies

270g oats
4 ripe bananas
3 tablespoons maple syrup
150g dried cranberries
4 red apples
2 teaspoons cinnamon

Preheat the oven to 200C.

Mash the bananas. Grate the apples and drain the liquid.

Mix all the ingredients together. Line a baking tray. Use one tablespoon of dough per cookie. Flatten each cookie.

Bake for half an hour, and allow to cool.

Cranberry and Pear Bake

1 cup dried cranberries
4 tablespoons pure maple syrup
5 ripe pears, cores and stems removed, and cut in quarters,
lengthwise
¼ cup pecans, chopped
Cinnamon

Preheat the oven to 175C.

Place the pears, cranberries and maple in a baking dish. Sprinkle with the cinnamon. Bake for 15 minutes, then stir. Sprinkle the nuts on top, and bake for another five minutes.

Quinoa Chocolate Cake

What I love about this cake is that it's so versatile. One week I'll make it with raspberries, and the next I'll use stem ginger or almond essence and decorate with almond flakes. It also lasts for a good few days in the refrigerator, too.

3 cups cooked quinoa (allow to cool)
1/3 cup rice or other plant milk
4 flax eggs
2 teaspoons pure vanilla extract
3/4 cup coconut oil, melted (or sunflower, if preferred)
1½ cups coconut sugar or raw brown sugar
1 cup unsweetened cocoa powder
1½ teaspoons baking powder
½ teaspoon bicarbonate of soda
½ teaspoon salt

Optional: punnet of fresh raspberries or blueberries, sugar-free fruit jam, flaked almonds

Preheat the oven to 180C. Lightly grease two round cake pans, and line the bottoms of the pans with parchment paper. Combine the milk, flax eggs and vanilla in a food processor. Process for a minute, then add the cooked quinoa and the coconut oil. Blend well until smooth.

In another bowl, whisk together the sugar, cocoa, baking powder, bicarbonate of soda and salt, then add to the quinoa mix. Mix well. Divide the batter in half between the two cake pans, then bake for 30 minutes.

Allow to cool for half an hour. Handle with care when

removing from the pans. Place your palm, with fingers outstretched, to hold the cake as you empty it from the pan.

When cooled, place the raspberries (or raspberry jam or frosting) between the two layers, if desired, and cover with frosting. Place in the fridge for two hours. Decorate with flowers and raspberries. This cake refrigerates beautifully, and will last a couple of days.

Frosting suggestion: combine a tub of plain vegan cream cheese with ½ cup cocoa powder and ½ cup coconut sugar and process until smooth. Spread over cake (once the cake has cooled).

Serve with cream or ice cream, if desired.

Apricot and Coconut Balls

It's not just carrots which are good for the eyes. Apricots are rich in vitamin A, too. Blessed to grow up in Australia, on 700 acres, I always marvelled at the wild apricot tree, just growing gracefully on its own. I never understood how or why it was there, but this I did know: No other apricots in the world ever came close, then or now, to the indescribably perfect nectar of the luscious fruit the tree so abundantly and generously proffered year after year.

1 cup oats
½ cup dried apricots
½ cup desiccated coconut
1 ripe banana
3 tablespoons maple syrup
2 tablespoons coconut oil
1 teaspoon vanilla extract

Process the oats, and then add the remaining ingredients. When well mixed, divide into balls and refrigerate for an hour or two.

Date and Pecan Balls

10 fresh Medjool dates, pitted
½ cup raw pecans
2 tablespoons cocoa
2 tablespoons desiccated coconut

Process the pecans and coconut until it resembles flour, then add the remaining ingredients. Form into golf-sized balls. Chill if desired.

Coconut and Pineapple Tropical Slice

Crust
1 cup almonds
1 cup Medjool dates
1 cup coconut oil, melted
1 cup desiccated coconut

Filling
400g silky tofu
1 cup coconut cream
½ cup maple syrup
1/3 cup coconut butter
3 tablespoons coconut oil
1/3 cup toasted coconut flakes
150g crushed pineapple (from a tin)

Line a cake tin with parchment paper.

Add all the ingredients for the crust together in a food processor and blend to combine. Press the mix into the bottom of the tin, and freeze.

Except for the coconut flakes, process the remaining ingredients, then gently pour over the crust. Sprinkle with coconut flakes.

Allow to set, ideally overnight in the fridge.

Vanilla Panna Cotta

4 tablespoons of agar flakes
2 cans coconut milk
Lemon zest
2 teaspoons vanilla
1 to 2 cups coconut sugar or maple syrup (depending on taste)

Gently heat the coconut milk and agar, stirring while it thickens.

Add the vanilla and lemon zest and the sweetener. Whisk to mix well. When thickened, place into glass serving jars and refrigerate overnight. Decorate with a few berries or make a small stew of your favourite fruits to serve alongside.

Courgette and Cranberry Cake

2½ cups Dove's Farm self-raising flour
1 tablespoon ground cinnamon
1 teaspoon salt
½ teaspoon ground nutmeg
Pinch of ground cloves
Pinch of ground ginger
500g courgettes, grated
1 cup coconut sugar
1 cup dried cranberries
4 flax eggs
¾ cup coconut or sunflower oil

Frosting
2 packs of Toffuti or other vegan cream cheese
1 cup coconut sugar (or more, to taste)
½ cup melted coconut oil
2 teaspoons vanilla extract
1 teaspoon lemon juice
Pinch of salt

Preheat oven to 180C. Line two sandwich cake tins with baking paper. Whisk the flour, cinnamon, nutmeg, salt, cloves and ginger together until combined. Combine the sugar and flax and mix until combined, then add the oil. Mix, and then add to a large bowl with the flour and courgettes. Stir through the cranberries. Bake for thirty minutes, and then leave in the cake tins for an hour before removing. Combine the frosting ingredients in a food processor and mix until smooth. Chill until ready to frost the (cooled) cake. If you can get hold of some natural pink food dye for the frosting, this makes a lovely touch to this cake.

Other Books By The Same Author

Fields of Lavender (poetry) 1991, out of print.

The Compassionate Years: history of the Royal New Zealand Society for the Protection of Animals, RNZSPCA 1993

The Drinks Are On Me: everything your mother never told you about breastfeeding (First edition published by Art of Change 2007) (Second edition by Starflower Press 2008)

Allattare Secondo Natura (Italian translation of The Drinks Are On Me 2009) published by Terra Nuova www.terranuovaedizioni.it

The Birthkeepers: reclaiming an ancient tradition (Starflower Press 2008)

Life Without School: the quiet revolution (Starflower Press 2010), co-authored by Paul, Bethany and Eliza Robinson

The Nurtured Family: ten threads of nurturing to weave through family life (Starflower Press 2011)

Natural Approaches to Healing Adrenal Fatigue (Starflower Press 2011)

Stretch Marks: selected articles from The Mother magazine 2002 – 2009, co-edited with Paul Robinson (Starflower Press)

The Mystic Cookfire: the sacred art of creating food for friends and family (more than 260 vegetarian recipes) (Starflower Press 2011)

The Blessingway: creating a beautiful Blessingway ceremony (Starflower Press 2012)

Baby Names Inspired by Mother Nature (Starflower Press 2012)

Cycle to the Moon: celebrating the menstrual trinity ~ menarche, menstruation, menopause (Starflower Press 2014)

I Create My Day (Starflower Press 2016)

Fiction
Mosaic (Starflower Press 2013)
Bluey's Cafe (Starflower Press 2013)
Blue Jeans (illustrated children's book) 2014 (out of print)
Sisters of the Silver Moon (2015) (book one, Gypsy Moon trilogy)
Behind Closed Doors (book two, Gypsy Moon trilogy) 2016

Upcoming in 2017:
Flowers in Her Hair (book three, Gypsy Moon trilogy)
Forever in Blue Jeans (republication of children's book, Blue Jeans)

About The Author

Veronika Sophia Robinson

The simple things in life bring Veronika enormous pleasure: Autumn leaves crunching under her feet, dewy cobwebs in the morning sunshine, the scent of earth after it rains, the sound of rain falling on a tin roof, sunrise and sunset, playful kittens, moonlight keeping her awake, ripe mangoes, her husband's kisses (not to mention his perfect coffee), her children's laughter, time with friends, gathering herbs and flowers from her garden, walking alone in the woods, birds circling on high, singing while she cooks food, intentional solitude, and cello music. She has two wonderful adult daughters (a musician and a writer), and a gorgeous granddaughter, and is happily married to her soulmate. Veronika is the author of eighteen books (fiction and non-fiction), and has been a celebrant since 1995. She officiates blessingways, namings, weddings, funerals, memorials, and other rites of passage. A second-generation astrologer, she had a successful international practice for thirteen years. Veronika loves bringing the archetypes and symbols of this divine language to use in a practical, life-affirming way. She has been studying metaphysics since childhood.

Instagram: veronika.robinson
Facebook: Love From My Kitchen (book) and
Veronika Sophia Robinson author and celebrant
Twitter: @veronikasophia #lovefrommykitchen
Pinterest: Veronika Robinson
www.veronikarobinson.com

About The Artist

Tracy Jane Roper

Tracy is passionate about art and its nourishment of the soul. Spending time in the woods with friends gives her the inspiration to create.

She is deeply rooted in Cornwall and its changing seasons, and juggles being a mama to two boys with the occasional days to further her love of art.

She also shares her passion with her children and her friends, and they regularly join in for messy fun.

Tracy is a keen cook, forager, home educator, animal lover, pagan and Nature geek, drawing on all these influences to create in her everyday life.

Find Tracy on Facebook at *WildLuna Art*.

Recipe Contents

Salads

Soups

Casseroles, bakes, roasts, lasagne and stews

Mediterranean Vegetables baked with lentils 86
Apricot and Black Bean Ragoût 87
Courgette and Aubergine Bake 88
Brazilian Bean Stew 90
Aubergine Curry 91
Macadamia and Red Pepper Roast 92
Beetroot-Jewelled Butternut Bake 93
Sunday Breakfast Lentils 95
Spaghetti and Meatballs 96
White Bean and Sage Roast 97
Sweet Potato and Brazil Nut Roast 98
Chestnut and Feta Roast 99
Mushroom Lasagne 100
Asparagus Lasagne 102
Mediterranean Vegetable Lasagne 103
Butternut and Sage Lasagne 104
Roast Fennel and Tomato Lasagne 106

Burgers, falafel, fritters and pizza
Mint and Pea Fritters 109
Herb and Almond Burgers 110
Fennel and Beetroot Croquettes 111
Carrot and Ginger Fritters 113
Irish Potato Cakes 115
Baked Black-Bean Falafel with Papaya and Mint Salsa 116
Sesame and Courgette Fritters 117
Garlicky Butternut Burgers 118
Sweet Potato and Red Onion Falafel 120
White Bean and Dill Burgers 121
Carrot and Nutmeg Fritters 122
Earthy Walnut and Lentil Burgers 123
Hash Browns for Eliza 125
Quinoa Pizza Crust 126
Socca Pizza 127
Polenta Pizza 128

Saucy stuff!
Smokey BBQ Sauce 131
White Bean and Cumin Hummus 131
Roast Pumpkin Seed And Nasturtium Pesto 132
Decadent Creamy Sauce 133
Sweet Ginger and Peanut Sauce 134
Rosemary Gravy 135

Voluptuous vegetables
Roast Cauliflower and Red Onion with Ginger and Peanut Butter Sauce 139
Marinated Picnic Vegetables 141
Mushroom-Stuffed Peppers 142
Butternut and Thyme Risotto 143

Mediterranean Vegetables with Mashed Butter Beans 144
Mushroom Pakoras 145
Asparagus with Mushroom Quinoa 147
Cheesy Cauliflower and Sesame Bites 148
Broccoli with Coconut and Peanut Cream 149
Courgette, Apple and Ginger Chutney 150
Thai Tofu with Noodles 151
Mushroom Tapenade 152
Sesame-Drenched Asparagus 153
Courgette Polenta Fries 154
My Heavenly Mushrooms 155
Corn and Cashew Dumplings with Mystic Masala Sauce 156
Beetroot and Walnut Risotto 158
Roast Cauliflower Tacos 159
Broccoli Pakora 160
Tandoori Roasted Cauliflower 161
Garlic-Maple Chantenay Carrots 162
Cauliflower and Date Pilaf 163

Sweets

Stewed Berry and Pear Crumble 166
Cranberry and Almond Slice 167
Carrot and Cinnamon Balls 168
Banana, Coconut and Chia Bread 169
Lemon and Coconut Rough and Tumble Cookies 170
Lime and Mango Cheesecake 171
Elderberry and Apple Crumble 173
Rhubarb and Citrus Crumble 174
Blueberry and Macadamia Crumble 175
No-Cook Raspberry and Pear Crumble 176
Raspberry and Vanilla-Infused Apple Crumble 177
Raspberry and White-Chocolate Cupcakes 178
Pear, Vanilla and Nutmeg Cake 179
Courgette and Chocolate Loaf 180
Apple and Cinnamon Cake 181
Passionfruit and Mango Cheesecake 182
Lemon and Coconut Cheesecake 183
Almond and Chocolate Chip Cookies 184
Banana Cookies 185
Cranberry and Pear Bake 186
Quinoa Chocolate Cake 187
Apricot and Coconut Balls 189
Date and Pecan Balls 189
Coconut and Pineapple Tropical Slice 190
Vanilla Panna Cotta 191
Courgette and Cranberry Cake 192

Lightning Source UK Ltd.
Milton Keynes UK
UKHW02f2002050618
323776UK00006B/594/P